Text Atlas of Practical Electrocardiography

T0190157

Massimo Romanò

Text Atlas of Practical Electrocardiography

A Basic Guide to ECG Interpretation

With contributions by Roberta Bertona

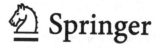 Springer

Massimo Romanò
Ospedale Civile di Vigevano
Vigevano
Italy

Translated from the Italian, with the author, by Marian Everett Kent

Chapters 7, 8, 9, 10, 12, 13, and 14 were written in collaboration with Dr. Roberta
Bertona of Vigevano Hospital

This is the English version of the Italian edition published under the title *Testo-atlante
di elettrocardiografia pratica*, © Springer-Verlag Italia 2009

ISBN 978-88-470-5740-1   ISBN 978-88-470-5741-8   (eBook)
DOI 10.1007/978-88-470-5741-8

Library of Congress Control Number: 2015933994

Springer Milan Heidelberg New York Dordrecht London
© Springer-Verlag Italia 2015

Printed on acid-free paper

Springer-Verlag Italia Srl. is part of Springer Science+Business Media (www.springer.com)

Preface

More than a century has passed since Willem Einthoven immersed his arms and legs in basins containing saline solution, connected them with wires to a galvanometer, and became the first man to record the electrical activity of the heart. For years, his "invention"—electrocardiography or ECG—was (along with the chest X-ray and a sensitive ear) the cornerstone of clinical cardiology. Generations of physicians have been fascinated and challenged by those messages in code, which to the trained and experienced eye revealed vast amounts of previously inaccessible information on the inner workings of the heart, information that could clearly improve the diagnosis, treatment, and prognosis of their patients.

Subsequent technological advances have sometimes overshadowed the decisive diagnostic role played by the ECG, but it has always maintained its status as an indispensable tool in a wide variety of settings, from the emergency rooms of small, rural hospitals to the sophisticated prehospital emergency service providers of teeming urban centers—in short, wherever human lives depend on the rapid recognition and proper treatment of acute coronary syndromes or life-threatening cardiac arrhythmias.

It's important to recall that the ECG should never be used as a replacement for clinical assessment: the tracings must first be analyzed in light of the clinical findings, described, and then used to formulate a diagnosis. How many patients have been diagnosed with ischemia solely on the bases of T wave inversion or nonspecific repolarization changes! This is what motivated me to create a concise text-atlas of electrocardiography based on no less than 30 years of experience as a hospital cardiologist, many of which were spent in frontier-hospitals, where clinicians find themselves face-to-face with a dismayingly complex array of major cardiac events in all of their various guises.

In a market that abounds with books and manuals on electrocardiography, the significance of this book lies primarily in its attempt to tie the fundamentals of electrophysiology to the variegated reality of clinical practice, abundantly illustrated with real-life ECG tracings. An essential handbook of sorts designed for rapid consultation by clinical cardiologists, emergency-department physicians and ambulance personnel, anesthesiologists involved in preoperative patient assessments, internists and intensivists caring for patients who are critically ill. With time (and years of study and experience and an undying awareness of one's own limits), each of these figures will come to regard the ECG as an indispensable resource for helping the patients in their care, an old but finely-honed diagnostic tool, which is almost quintessentially patient-centered and at the same time completely "at home" in the sophisticated, high-tech world of modern medicine. (One of the many examples that come to mind—and are explored in detail in the book—is the interventional cardiology lab, where the ECG tracings recorded during coronary angioplasty are indispensable for verifying the success of revascularization and rapidly detecting complications.)

Special thanks go first of all to my patients, who have taught me so much (often much more than I realized at the time); to the colleagues and co-workers who have helped me collect the numerous tracings included in the volume; to my co-author Dr. Roberta Bertona, for her valuable contributions, untiring support, meticulous attention to detail, and lively intelligence; to Drs. Madeleine Hofmann and Donatella Rizza of Springer-Verlag, who believed in and supported this project from the very start; and to Drs. Catherine Mazars and Angela Vanegas for their assistance and patience in the realization of this project.

And last but not least, to my mentor, Prof. Ugo Garbarini, *Maestro di Medicina* at the University of Milan: along with the fundamentals of my profession, he instilled in me an unwavering and broad-ranging fascination with the "language" of electrocardiography: from the esthetics of its waveforms—rhythmic, almost musical—to the remarkable eloquence, subtlety, and expressive range of the statements they make about the heart and the body in general. Without these foundations, this book would never have been possible.

Vigevano, Italy   Massimo Romanò
February 2015

Acronyms and Abbreviations

AF	Atrial fibrillation
AFL	Atrial flutter
AIVR	Accelerated idioventricular rhythm
AMI	Acute myocardial infarction
AVN	Atrioventricular node
AVB	Atrioventricular blocks
AVRT	Atrioventricular reentrant tachycardia
AVNRT	Atrioventricular nodal reentrant tachycardia
bpm	Beats per minute
BBB	Bundle-branch block
CTI	Cavotricuspid isthmus
DC	Direct-current
ECG	Electrocardiogram
IC-ECG	Intracardiac electrocardiogram
LAD	Left anterior descending artery
LAFB	Left anterior fascicular block
LBBB	Left bundle-branch block
LCx	Left circumflex artery
LPFB	Left posterior fascicular block
MI	Myocardial infarction
NSTEMI	Non-ST-segment-elevation myocardial infarction
PTCA	Percutaneous transluminal coronary angioplasty
PJRT	Permanent reciprocating junctional tachycardia
PM	Pacemaker
RBBB	Right bundle-branch block
RCA	Right coronary artery
SA	Sinoatrial
STEMI	ST-segment-elevation myocardial infarction
SVEB	Supraventricular ectopic beats
SVT	Supraventricular tachycardia
TdP	Torsade de pointes
VEB	Ventricular ectopic beats
VT	Ventricular tachycardia
WPW	Wolff-Parkinson-White

Contents

General Principles of Anatomy and Cellular Electrophysiology

An Anatomical Overview of the Excitation-Conduction System of the Heart

The electrical activity of the heart is governed by the sinoatrial (SA) node (also known as the node of Keith and Flack) (Fig. 1.1), a microscopic structure located in the right atrium, at the junction between the atrium and the superior vena cava. It is made of pacemaker cells, which are intrinsically capable of generating rhythmic electrical impulses at rates that normally range from 60 to 100 beats per minute (bpm). The electrical current that originates here is propagated to the atria along preformed pathways known as the internodal tracts: the anterior internodal tract (known as Bachmann's bundle), which includes a branch for the left atrium; the middle internodal tract (Wenckebach's bundle); and the posterior internodal tract (Thorel's bundle).

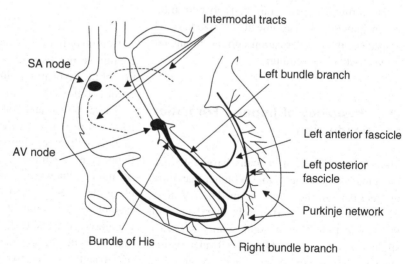

Fig. 1.1 The anatomy of the conduction system. *SA* sinoatrial, *AV* atrioventricular. See text for details

SA node

Intermodal tracts

Left bundle branch

Left anterior fascicle

AV node

Left posterior fascicle

Purkinje network

Bundle of His

Right bundle branch

M. Romanò, *Text Atlas of Practical Electrocardiography*,
DOI 10.1007/978-88-470-5741-8_1, © Springer-Verlag Italia 2015

From the atria, the depolarization wave spreads to the atrioventricular (AV) node (or node of Tawara), the second fundamental station in the heart's electrical conduction system. It is located in the posteroinferior region of the interatrial septum near the opening of the coronary sinus and represents the only normal connection between the atria and the ventricles. It is therefore the obligatory point of passage for impulses travelling to the ventricles.

Propagation of the electrical impulses from the AV node to the ventricles themselves occurs through a specialized conduction system. The proximal portion, which is known as the bundle of His, begins at the AV node and then divides within the ventricular septum to form the right and left bundle branches. The right bundle branch continues down the right side of the septum, just beneath the endocardium, and at the base of the anterior papillary muscle in the right ventricle, it divides again, sending fibers to the free wall of the right ventricle and to the left side of the septum. The left bundle branch, which is larger in caliber than the right, divides to form an anterior fascicle, which supplies the wall of the left ventricle, and an posterior fascicle, which supplies the left side of the septum. The two bundle branches continue to divide, forming a densely ramified subendocardial system known as the Purkinje fiber network, which propagates the depolarization current throughout the ventricular myocardium.

The Physiology of Impulse Formation and Conduction

The SA node has an intrinsic discharge rate (normal range: 60–100 bpm) that is higher than those of other parts of the myocardium. The AV node, which is the most important subsidiary station in the conduction system, emits impulses at a slightly lower rate (40–60 bpm). Under normal and pathological conditions, other portions of the conduction system or even the ordinary working myocardium are capable of firing at rates ranging from 20 to 40 bpm (Fig. 1.2).

Cardiac automaticity

Primary pacemaker
–NSA 60-100 bpm

Subsidiary pacemakers
Atria ~ 60 bpm
AV node 40-60 bpm
His-Purkinje system
30-40 bpm
Ventricles <30 bpm

Fig. 1.2 The hierarchy of cardiac pacemakers. *Asterisks* indicate areas of the myocardium itself that are potential ectopic foci

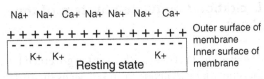

Resting potential of the cell = –90 mV

Fig. 1.3 The resting action potential of the cardiomyocytes. The outer surface of the cell membrane is positively charged, due to the high concentration of sodium and calcium ions. The intracellular compartment is characterized by high concentration of potassium ions, which renders the inner surface of the membrane electronegative

Contraction of the heart is regulated by a continuous process of repetitive electrical excitation of the myocardium in which every electrical event is followed by a mechanical event.

The electrical and contractile activities of the heart are mediated by the constant flow of ions (mainly sodium, calcium, and potassium) through lipoprotein structures in the cardiomyocyte cell membrane known as ion channels. If microelectrodes were placed on both sides of this membrane, it would show that, under resting conditions, the inside of the cell has a negative charge while the outside is positively charged. The result is a negative resting transmembrane potential of approximately −90 millivolts) (Fig. 1.3). The potential reflects the existence of ion concentration gradients across the membrane characterized by high levels of sodium outside the cell and high potassium levels in the intracellular compartment. The gradients are maintained by active transmembrane transport systems (the ATPase-dependent sodium/potassium pump).

The resting action potential of the cell membrane is modified by a rapid influx of sodium ions from the extracellular compartment, an event referred to as *depolarization* (Fig. 1.4), because it reverses the membrane's polarity (the inner surface becomes positive, the outer surface negative). The electrical phenomena that occur when the cell is activated in this manner are referred to collectively as the *action potential*, and they can be recorded, as shown in Fig. 1.5. The rapid inward current of sodium ions corresponds to Phase 0 of the action potential. It is followed by:

– Phase 1, during which the influx of Sodium ions slows, the transmembrane action potential is about 0 millivolts (mV), and there is a transient outflow of potassium;

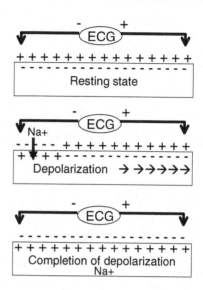

Fig. 1.4 The flow of sodium ions into the cell depolarizes the cell membrane, reversing its polarity, which is now characterized by extracellular negativity and intracellular positivity. *ECG* electrocardiogram

Fig. 1.5 Diagram of the resting transmembrane action potential and its phases. See text for details

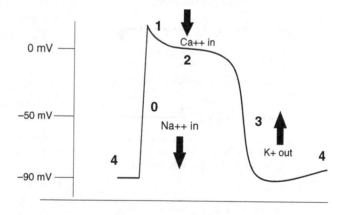

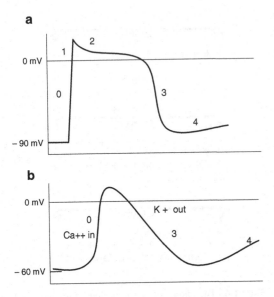

Fig. 1.6 Diagrams of (**a**) the sodium-dependent action potential of the atrial and ventricular myocardial cells (see text for details), and (**b**) the calcium-dependent action potential of the pacemaker cells (SA and AV nodes). See text for details

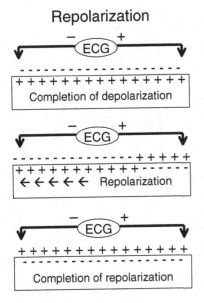

Fig. 1.7 In the repolarization phase, the original polarity of the cell membrane (positive outside, negative inside) is restored. *ECG* electrocardiogram

– Phase 2, which is characterized by a slow inward-directed flow of calcium ions that triggers the release of intracellular stores of calcium, which bind to the contractile proteins of the cardiomyocytes.
– Phase 3, which marks the beginning of repolarization, is produced by a biphasic (initially rapid, then slow) outflow of potassium ions, which continues until the resting electrical potential of the membrane has been restored;
– Phase 4, during which the resting negative polarity is maintained by an outward flow of sodium ions and an inward flow of potassium ions.

There are two main types of action potential:
– the fast sodium-dependent action potential, which is characterized by a rapid phase-0-upstroke and is typical of the cells in the His-Purkinje system and those of the atrial and ventricular myocardium (Fig. 1.6a);
– the slow, calcium-dependent action potential, which is typical of the cells of the SA and AV nodes and of ischemic myocardial cells (Fig. 1.6b). Phase 0 of the slow potential is mainly related to the entry of calcium ions. The resting action potential of the slow fibers is less electronegative than that of the fast cells (− 60 mV vs. −90 mV). Phase 0 is also slower, with a more gradual upstroke, and the speed of conduction is proportionally reduced.

Phase 4 is an unstable phase characterized by progressive, spontaneous depolarization of the cell membrane. This phenomenon, which is known as *automaticity*, is a potential property of all the cardiac cells. It is normally displayed primarily by the SA and AV nodes and the His-Purkinje system, but under certain circumstances, the atrial and ventricular myocardium can also exhibit spontaneous automaticity. After the cell has been depolarized, its initial electrical status is restored via the phenomenon known as repolarization (Fig. 1.7).

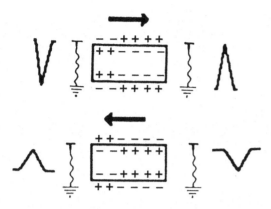

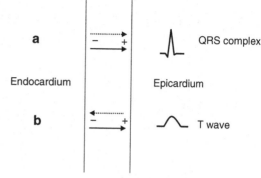

Fig. 1.8 Depolarization and repolarization. *Upper diagram*: Electrical activation of the cell with inversion of the transmembrane polarity. This generates a flow of current to areas still in the resting state. The *arrow* indicates the depolarization vector. *Lower diagram*: Repolarization proceeds in the opposite direction. Leads attached to the extremities record vectors as positive (wavefronts travelling toward the electrode) or negative (wavefronts travelling away from the electrode) deflections

Fig. 1.9 Direction of the depolarization process-QRS complex (**a**) and of the repolarization process-T wave (**b**) through the myocardial wall from the endocardium to the epicardium. The two phases are characterized by opposite polarities and directions. Therefore, the orientations of the two vectors are the same

As noted above, application of an electrical stimulus to the cell membrane reverses its polarity (depolarization). Current then flows from the activated (depolarized) cell toward contiguous cells that are still in the resting state (Fig. 1.8). The flow of current between cells with different electrical states creates a dipole, which is simply a pair of electric charges of equal magnitude but opposite polarity. The dipole can be represented as a vector, which is characterized by *length* (reflecting the magnitude of its electrical charges in millivolts), *direction* (determined by the predominant depolarization wavefronts in the given region and phase), and *orientation*. Conventionally, the tail of the vector is designated as negative (i.e., already activated) and the head (the zone still not activated) as positive.

Depolarization of the myocardial cells proceeds from the endocardium towards the epicardium. The subendocardial cells, which are depolarized, are thus electronegative relative to the epicardial cells, which are still polarized. The direction of the depolarization vector (complex QRS) therefore has the same orientation as that of the depolarization wave. The corresponding ECG leads record a positive deflection. Repolarization proceeds in the opposite direction to that of depolarization: the subepicardial cells repolarize first and are thus electropositive relative to the subendocardial cells. Therefore, the orientation of the dipole corresponding to the repolarization vector (the T-wave) is the same as that of the depolarization vector (Fig. 1.9).

This current flow is capable of depolarizing other cells in the vicinity in a chain reaction that spreads through the entire myocardium: the events that ensue can be recorded at the body surface and represented graphically as a succession of positive and negative deflections, the ECG.

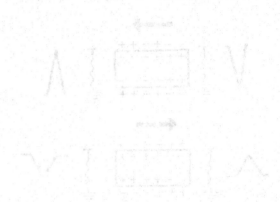

The Electrocardiographic Leads

2

As noted in Chap. 1, propagation of the electrical stimulus in the heart can be represented as dipoles. For simplicity's sake, each dipole is represented as a vector with a negatively charged tail and a positively charged head (Fig. 2.1). ECG electrodes are attached to the surfaces of specific body areas and connected to one another to form leads. The electrical potentials in the heart are recorded by the leads and transmitted them to the electrocardiograph, which is a galvanometric recording device (Fig. 2.2). Vectors travelling away from the recording point are represented by negative deflections; those moving toward the recording point appear as positive waves (Fig. 2.3).

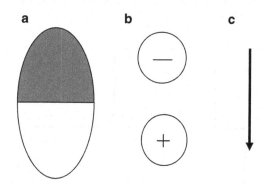

Fig. 2.1 (a) A partially depolarized myocardial fiber (*gray area*); (b) a dipole; and (c) a vector with a negative tail and positive head

Fig. 2.2 Electrodes attached to the right and left arms or legs are connected to a galvanometer to record the ECG, by means of a lead

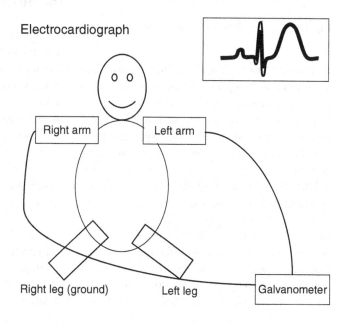

M. Romanò, *Text Atlas of Practical Electrocardiography*,
DOI 10.1007/978-88-470-5741-8_2, © Springer-Verlag Italia 2015

A vector moving toward the exploring electrode produces a positive deflection on ECG

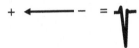

A vector moving away from the exploring electrode produces a negative deflection on ECG

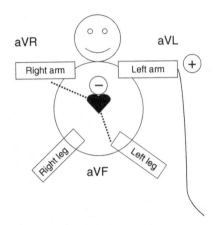

Fig. 2.5 Diagram of the Goldberger augmented limb leads with a sample recording from lead aVL (*solid line*). The right arm and left leg are "short-circuited" to produce a reference electrode, which is ideally located in the center of the chest and has a potential of zero (*dotted line*). The aVR and aVF leads are recorded in a similar manner, short-circuiting the other leads in rotation

Fig. 2.3 The *upper vector*, which is moving toward the electrode, produces a positive deflection. The *lower vector* moving away from the electrode produces a negative deflection

exploring (or positive) electrode records voltage at one site relative to an electrode with zero potential, which is ideally located over the center of the heart. The zero potential is achieved by joining the nonexploring electrodes to a central terminal known as the Wilson central terminal (Fig. 2.5).

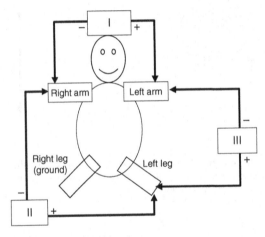

Fig. 2.4 Diagram of the bipolar limb leads. See text for details

The standard leads include three bipolar limb leads and nine "unipolar" leads, three limb leads and six precordial leads. Each bipolar lead records the difference between the electrical potentials detected by two electrodes, one positive, the other negative, placed on two different points of the body surface (Fig. 2.4). If the potential difference detected by the positive electrode is greater than that detected by the negative electrode, the electrocardiograph records an upward (or positive) deflection. If the positive electrode detects a smaller potential difference is smaller than that detected by the negative electrode, a downward or negative deflection will be recorded. As for the so-called unipolar leads, the

The Bipolar Limb Leads

The bipolar limb leads—I, II, and III—record the potential difference between two points of observation (the right arm, the left arm, and the left leg), one connected to the positive electrode, the other to the negative electrode. The left arm is conventionally considered positive relative to the right arm and negative with respect to the left leg, while the left leg is considered positive relative to the right arm. The ground electrode is conventionally placed on the right leg (Fig. 2.4). The connection of the limb leads is as follows:
- Lead I: left arm (+), right arm (−)
- Lead II: left leg (+), right arm (−)
- Lead III: left leg (+), left arm (−).

Graphically linked, the three limb leads form a triangle (Einthoven's triangle), whose center is ideally the heart (Fig. 2.6).

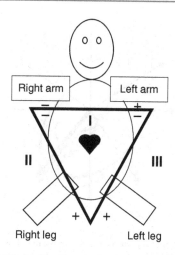

Fig. 2.6 The bipolar limb leads and Einthoven's triangle

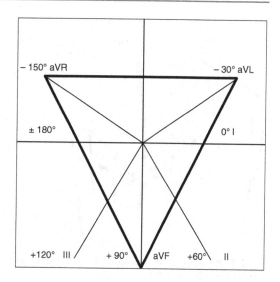

Fig. 2.7 The hexaxial reference system: Positions of the bipolar and unipolar limb leads superimposed on Einthoven's triangle. See text for details

The Augmented "Unipolar" Limb Leads

The bipolar leads record the potential difference between two limbs. The so-called unipolar leads (limb and precordial) consist of pairs of electrodes (and for this reason, there is some debate about whether they should actually be referred to as unipolar), although in this case, the pairs are *derived*. They include a single positive electrode placed on a limb or on the chest and a zero reference electrode, which is a combination of the three limb electrodes. With the reference electrode connected to the negative pole of the electrocardiograph, the positive or exploring electrodes can detect *absolute* variations in the electrical potential from various angles (Fig. 2.5).

Like their bipolar counterparts, the unipolar limb leads use electrodes attached to the right and left arms and the left leg. The electrodes that record the variations in potential are located at the vertices of the triangle of Einthoven, that is, on the right shoulder (aVR, R=right), the left shoulder (aVL, L=left), and the left hip (aVF,

F=foot). The "aV" in these terms stands for "augmented voltage." In fact, the potentials recorded in this manner are small in amplitude and must therefore be artificially amplified.

The relations between the bipolar and unipolar limb leads are diagramed in what is known as the hexaxial system (Fig. 2.7). To facilitate correct placement, the electrodes are often color-coded. In Europe, red is used for the right arm, black for the right leg, yellow for the left arm, and green for the left leg. In the United States, white is used for the right arm, green for the right leg, black for the left arm, and red for the left leg.

The Unipolar Precordial Leads

The exploring electrodes of the precordial leads are placed on conventional points of the chest (Fig. 2.8), and the theoretical zero reference electrode is the same one is used in the unipolar limb leads. These leads detect vectors that are active in the horizontal plane of the heart.

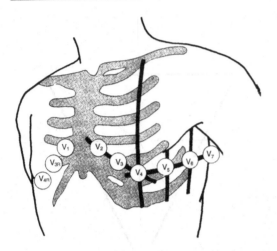

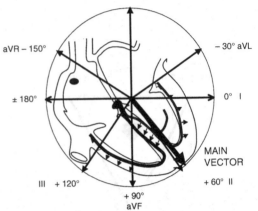

Fig. 2.8 Positions of the precordial leads. See text for details From Slavich, 1997

Fig. 2.9 Frontal plane of the heart visualized by the limb leads. Each lead analyzes the heart from a different point of view: Leads II, III, and aVF depict activity in the inferior wall, leads I and aVL the lateral wall, and lead aVR explores the atrioventricular orifices

There are six standard precordial leads:
- V1: the electrode is placed in the fourth intercostal space, on the right sternal border
- V2: electrode in the fourth intercostal space, on the left sternal border
- V3: electrode placed midway between V2 and V4
- V4: electrode placed in the fifth intercostal space, on the anterior midclavicular line
- V5: electrode is horizontally aligned with V4, on the anterior axillary line
- V6: electrode placed on the midaxillary line and aligned horizontally with V4.
  Additional leads can also be used, such as:
- V7: electrode placed on the posterior axillary line at the same level as V4
- V8: electrode placed at the left scapular angle, at the same level as V4
- V9: electrode in the paravertebral region at the same level as V4
- V3R and V4R, electrodes placed to the right of the sternum, at the same levels as V3 and V4.

Each lead analyzes the heart from a different point of view. Leads II, III, and aVF depict activity in the inferior wall, leads I and aVL monitor the left lateral wall, and lead aVR views the atrioventricular orifices. (The impulse travels away from these orifices and spreads from the base to the apex of the heart.

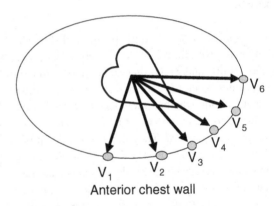

Fig. 2.10 The precordial leads view electrical activity in the horizontal plane

Consequently, lead aVR is nearly always negative.) (Fig. 2.9). Precordial leads V1 through V3 explore the activation of the right ventricle and the interventricular septum; V4 explores that of the apex, and V5 and V6 record activation of the lateral wall. Leads V7 through V9 record activity in the posterolateral wall, and leads V3R and V4R record that of the right ventricle (Fig. 2.10).

Table 2.1 shows the steps that should be followed to ensure correct recording and interpretation of the ECG.

Table 2.1 Check-list for performing an electrocardiogram

1. Collect necessary equipment and supplies:
   a. Ten electrodes connected to the recording cable of the electrocardiograph.
   b. Alcohol (for cleaning the skin).
2. Prepare the patient:
   a. Use alcohol to remove oils from the skin of the wrists, ankles, and chest. Men's chests should be shaved to remove body hair and facilitate the placement of electrodes.
   b. Attach the electrodes (see text).
3. Record the electrocardiographic tracing:
   a. Make sure that the paper speed is set at 25 mm/sec;
   b. For each group of leads (3 or 6 depending on the type of electrocardiograph), press the calibration button to make sure it is set at 10 mV (or that this setting is reflected in the calibration signal that appears on the paper);
   c. Begin recording with the bipolar limb leads (I, II, and III) followed by the augmented limb leads (aVR, aVL, aVF). Next record the standard precordial leads (V1 through V6) and when necessary the additional precordial leads.
4. After the recording has been completed, wash the electrodes and turn the electrocardiograph off. (Make sure the machine is attached to an AC power source to keep the battery charged.). Proper maintenance of the electrocardiograph is indispensable to ensure high-quality recordings.

The Normal Electrocardiogram

3

The electrocardiograph is a galvanometer calibrated to produce a deflection with an amplitude of 1 cm for every millivolt (mV) of voltage. The electrocardiogram (ECG) is recorded on graph paper divided into small 1-mm squares. At the standard paper speed of 25 mm/s, each small square corresponds to 40 ms (Fig. 3.1). Before the ECG is recorded, the machine must be calibrated to ensure that it is functioning correctly, and the square (or rectangular) calibration mark must be recorded on the tracing.

Fig. 3.1 Single components of an ECG and their temporal relations

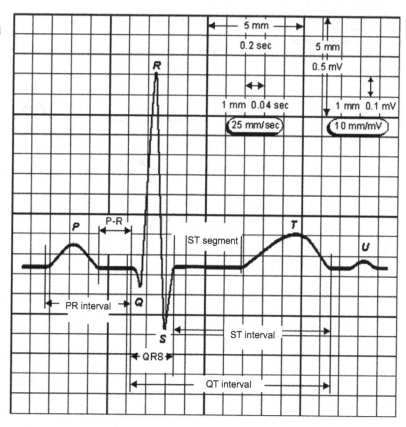

M. Romanò, *Text Atlas of Practical Electrocardiography*,
DOI 10.1007/978-88-470-5741-8_3, © Springer-Verlag Italia 2015

The ECG is composed of a series of deflections, the P wave, the QRS complex, and the T wave, separated by isoelectric segments known as the PR interval and the ST segment.

The P Wave

The P wave is the graphic representation of atrial electrical activation. It normally has a duration of 50–120 ms and a maximum amplitude of 2.5 millimeters (generally recorded in lead II). Atrial depolarization normally proceeds downward from the SA node and from right to left. The mean electrical axis in the frontal plane thus ranges from +10° to +90°. The P wave is positive in the inferior leads, negative in lead aVR, and positive in all the precordial leads except V1, where it is biphasic (positive, then negative). Deviations from these norms are suggestive of an ectopic atrial rhythm. The P wave includes two components: the first corresponds to the activation of the right atrium, the second to that of the left atrium. The phase of atrial repolarization—the Ta wave or complex—is normally not visible on surface ECGs: it occurs during ventricular depolarization and is therefore obscured by the QRS complex (Fig. 3.2).

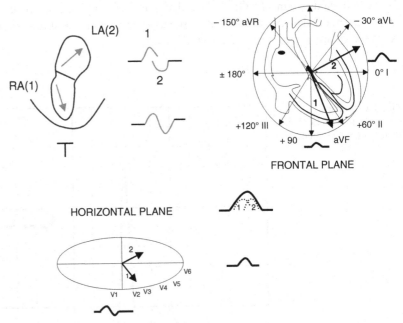

Fig. 3.2 The P wave is composed of two main vectors, which reflect depolarization of the right (1) and left (2) atria. The two vectors are shown in the frontal plane (as viewed by the limb leads) and in the horizontal plane (as seen by the precordial leads). *RA* right atrium, *LA* left atrium

The PR Interval

The PR interval represents the time needed for atrioventricular conduction. It is measured from the beginning of atrial activation to the beginning of ventricular activation, and its normal duration is from 120 to 200 ms.

The QRS Complex

The QRS complex represents ventricular depolarization, which begins in the interventricular septum, proceeding from the endocardium to the epicardium and from left to right. It then extends to the free anterior walls and finally the posterobasal regions of the two ventricles (Fig. 3.3). The main direction of the depolarization wavefront is from top to bottom and from right to left in the frontal plane and from back to front and from right to left in the horizontal plane. In the frontal plane, the electrical axis of the QRS complex generally ranges from −10° to +80°.

The normal QRS complex has a duration of 60–100 ms. The Q wave is the first negative deflection after the P wave, the R wave is the

Fig. 3.3 Ventricular depolarization. Phase 1 involves depolarization of the interventricular septum; phase 2 that of the free wall of the ventricles; and phase 3 that of the posterobasal wall

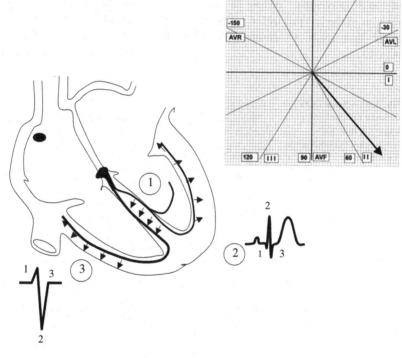

first positive deflection, and S wave is the first negative deflection after the R wave. A second positive deflection sometimes follows the S wave and is indicated by the letter R'. Upper- and lower-case letters are used to designate high- and low-voltage waves, respectively. The amplitude of the QRS complex varies: aside from cardiac diseases, it is affected by the size of the chest and the volume of air interposed between the heart and the exploring electrodes. The maximum amplitudes of the R wave are <23 mm in the frontal plane (usually seen in lead II) and <25 mm in leads V5 and V6. The maximum amplitude of the S wave in V2 is <25 mm. A normal Q wave is characterized by an amplitude that is less than 25 % of that of the R wave that follows it and measures <3 mm in the left precordial leads and ≤2 mm in the limb leads. Its duration should be less than 40 ms.

In the precordial leads, the R-wave amplitude increases progressively from lead V1 to lead V5, while that of the S wave decreases, a phenomenon referred to as R-wave progression. The amplitudes of the two waves generally become similar in lead V3 or V4 (i.e., the R/S ratio becomes ~1). The point where this occurs is referred to as the transition zone (Fig. 3.4), and in some healthy individuals, it appears earlier, i.e., in lead V2 or V3. This normal variant is referred to as clockwise rotation around an ideal longitudinal axis, which passes through the heart from the plane of the atrioventricular valves to the apex (Fig. 3.5). In leads V5 and V6, the interval between the beginning of the QRS complex and the peak of the R wave normally does not exceed 40 ms (in the absence of a Q wave) or 50 ms (if a recordable Q wave is present). This interval, which is known as the R-wave peak time, reflects epicardial depolarization of the ventricles.

Fig. 3.4 Normal ECG showing the zone of transition in R wave progression between leads V3 and V4

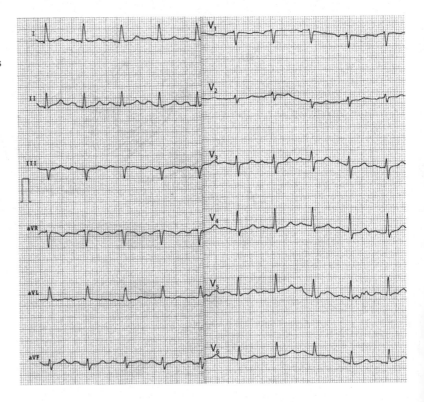

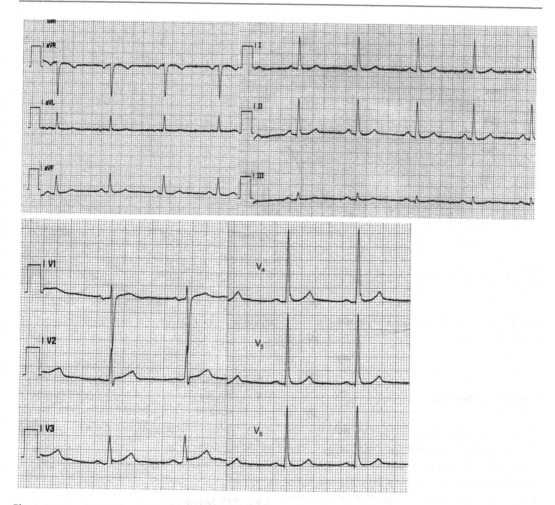

Fig. 3.5 Normal ECG characterized by electrical clockwise rotation around the longitudinal axis, which is reflected by the appearance of the QRS transition zone in V2-V3

The J Point

The J point corresponds to the end of ventricular depolarization. It is located between the end of QRS complex and the beginning of the ST segment, generally on the isoelectric line.

The T Wave

The phase of ventricular repolarization includes the ST segment and the T wave. The latter has asymmetric ascending and descending limbs and tends to be positive in the extremity leads (except aVR) and in the precordial leads (except V1). In

rare cases, the T wave is followed by a U wave, which is usually positive. Its significance is controversial.

The ST Segment

The ST segment is measured from the J point to the onset of the T wave, and it usually remains close to the isoelectric line. Mild ST segment depression (less than 0.5 mm) is not considered pathological. Elevations of up to 1–2 mm, especially in leads V2 and V3, may also be nonpathological, particularly in patients with increased vagal tone (Fig. 3.6).

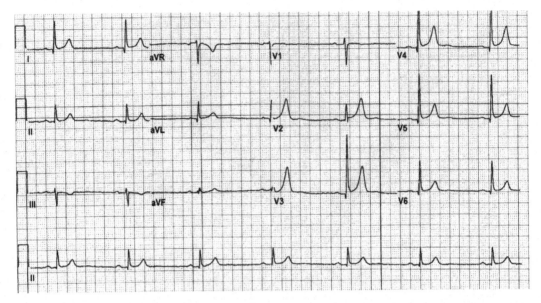

Fig. 3.6 ECG in a healthy subject with marked sinus bradycardia, a short QT interval, and upward concave ST segment elevation, elements typical of increased vagal tone

The QT Interval

The QT interval corresponds to electrical systole, that is, the interval from the beginning of ventricular depolarization to the end of repolarization. Its duration is inversely proportional to the heart rate. The rate-corrected QT interval [QTc] can be calculated with the Bazett formula, where:

$$QTc = QT/\sqrt{RR'}$$

where R–R' is the number of seconds between two consecutive QRS complexes. In adults, the QTc is normally less than 440 ms.

In young, healthy subjects, the QT interval may be short and associated with bradycardia owing to the predominance of the parasympathetic nervous system. Nonpathological ST-segment elevation may also be present in these cases (Fig. 3.6). It represents "early repolarization" caused by increased vagal tone and can be distinguished from pathological elevation (that associated with myocardial infarction or acute pericarditis—see sections on these disorders) in part by its bowl-shaped configuration (upward concavity). To this end, it may be useful to measure the ST segment/T wave ratio.

The height of the ST-segment elevation (in millimeters) is divided by the peak height of the T wave. A ratio of <0.25 is suggestive of early repolarization; a higher ratio is indicative of pericarditis.

The TQ Interval

This interval is measured from the end of the T wave to the beginning of the QRS complex. It corresponds to the phase of electrical diastole, and its importance will be discussed in Chap. 11, which deals with ischemic heart disease.

The Electrical Axis

The electrical axis of the heart is the spatial orientation of its mean vector, that is, the sum of the individual vectors of the various ECG components, mainly the P wave and QRS complex. The mean vector originates at the center of Einthoven's triangle. The six limb leads explore the heart along its frontal axis. The hexaxial reference system shown in Fig. 3.7 is used to

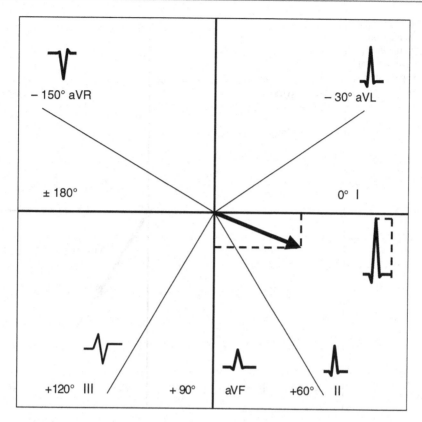

Fig. 3.7 The hexaxial system constructed with the limb leads. The diagram is used to identify the electrical axis in the frontal plane. Each lead is represented by a line whose continuous portion constitutes the projection on the frontal plane. Lead I is conventionally designated as the point with an angle of 0°. In contrast, each vector that moves away from zero in an upward, counterclockwise direction marks a decrease up to −180°

determine the orientation of the cardiac vectors in the frontal plane. The standard and augmented limb leads are mapped onto a diagram so that they intersect at a common point at the center of the heart and aVF, aVR, and aVL are perpendicular to leads I, II, and III, respectively. The mean atrial and ventricular depolarization vectors—clinically, the most useful—are identified respectively as the axes of the P wave and the QRS complex. Identifying the direction of the mean electrical axis provides insight into the morphology of the tracings obtained with each limb lead and makes it possible to identify certain electrocardiographic abnormalities, such as hemiblocks.

Two fundamental concepts need to be recalled when calculating the electrical axis of a vector:

1. Vectors moving toward the exploring electrode produce positive deflections; those moving away from the exploring electrode produce negative deflections.
2. A vector lying perpendicular to the exploring electrode produces no deflection (i.e., an isoeletric line) or an isobiphasic complex consisting of two consecutive deflections of opposite polarity.

To calculate the electrical axis, one identifies the lead in which the vector is most positive, the one in which it is most negative, and the one in which it produces a isobiphasic complex.

Normally, the mean electrical axis of the P wave is usually +60° (range: +10° to +90°); that of the QRS is +60° (range: −10° to +80°), and that of the T wave +40° (range: −10° to +70°) (Fig. 3.8).

Fig. 3.8 Calculation of the electrical axis in the frontal plane: normally, the mean axis of the P wave and that of the QRS complex are both around +60°

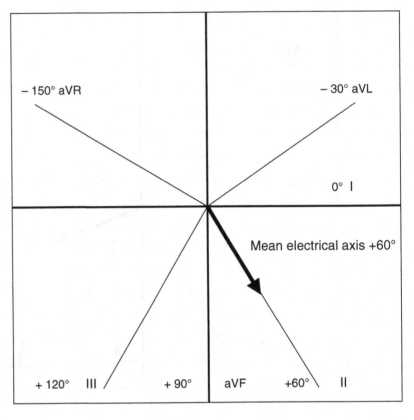

Interpreting the ECG

When reading an ECG, it is important to use a systematic approach designed to correctly identify abnormalities involving the various components. This approach includes the analysis of:

1. heart rate
2. rhythm (including measurement of the duration of the various intervals);
3. the electrical axes of the P wave and the QRS complex (Fig. 3.8).
4. the amplitudes of the P wave, the QRS complex, and the T wave;
5. the morphology of the P wave, the QRS complex, the ST segment, and the T wave.

If the rhythm is regular, the simplest way to calculate heart rate is with the so-called Rule of 300 (Fig. 3.9). The number of squares between consecutive P waves (for atrial rates) or consecutive R waves (for ventricular rates) are counted. Each small square represents 40 milliseconds, which means that 1500 small squares (or 300 large squares) represent 1 minute. The number of squares between consecutive complexes is then divided by 300 to obtain the rate in beats per minute (bpm).

Fig. 3.9 Calculating the heart rate with the Rule of 300. The rate in this case is around 38 bpm. See text for details

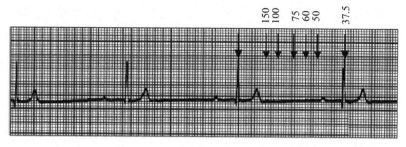

A simple approach to the reading of an ECG tracing (discussed at length later) involves the following series of questions:

1. Is there any electrical activity? (This may seem like an odd way to start, but it is essential. Lack of activity when the patient is conscious suggests that the electrocardiograph is not working or the leads have not been properly connected; in an unconscious patient, it might reflect asystole.)

2. Is the rhythm of the QRS complexes regular or irregular?

3. What is the ventricular rate? (See text for calculation.)

4. Is the width (i.e., the duration) of the QRS complex normal or increased?

5. Is there detectable atrial activity?

6. What kind of correlation is there between the atrial and ventricular activity?

Electrical Bases of the Arrhythmias

Arrhythmias are cardiac rhythm abnormalities, that is, rhythms differing from the normal sinus rhythm, which is characterized by heart rates ranging from 60 to 100 beats per minute (bpm). When the rate falls below 60 bpm, the patient is said to have a bradyarrhythmia, whereas rates above 100 bpm are referred to as tachyarrhythmias. Electrocardiographic analysis of an arrhythmia is not limited, however, to heart rate (increased versus decreased): it also includes the rhythm (which can be regular or irregular), the origin (supraventricular versus ventricular), and the morphology of the QRS complex (narrow versus wide) (Table 4.1).

Arrhythmias can be caused by any of the following:

1. abnormal impulse formation;
2. abnormal impulse conduction;
3. both of the above mechanisms.

Bradyarrhythmias are the result of delayed or absent formation and/or conduction of the impulse at any level of the conduction system (Fig. 4.1).

Three electrophysiological mechanisms give rise to tachyarrhythmias: abnormal automaticity, the reentry phenomenon, and triggered activity.

The first involves increased spontaneous firing by pacemaker cells or common cardiomyocytes. It can be caused by various factors, including increased sympathetic activity, ischemia, acidosis, and hypokalemia. These conditions are characterized by increases in the slope of phase 4 of the action potential and in the firing rate of the cardiac cells (Fig. 4.2).

The second (and most common) mechanism is that of reentry. Three conditions must be met before reentry can occur (Fig. 4.3). First, the electrical stimulus reaches a closed circuit, anatomical or functional, which consists of two pathways with different conduction velocities and refractory periods. Second, one of the two pathways presents a unidirectional block, and third, the second pathway is characterized by delayed electrical conduction. Reentry occurs when a premature ectopic impulse (a prerequisite for arrhythmia onset) is travelling along the usual conduction pathways and encounters the two electrophysiologically distinct pathways of the circuit. One offers slow conduction but a relatively short refractory period, which means it can be reexcited fairly early; the other pathway offers more rapid conduction but it remains refractory (and therefore cannot be re-excited) for a longer period of time. Anterograde transmission of the ectopic impulse along the "fast" pathway is blocked because its fibers are still refractory. In contrast, the short refractory period of the "slow" pathway is over, and the impulse can use this route to proceed on its course. If conduction

M. Romanò, *Text Atlas of Practical Electrocardiography*,
DOI 10.1007/978-88-470-5741-8_4, © Springer-Verlag Italia 2015

Table 4.1 Criteria for ECG assessment of arrhythmias

Heart rate (bradyarrhythmias: rate <60 bpm; tachyarrhythmias: rate >100 bpm)

Rhythm (regular or irregular)

Origin (supraventricular vs. ventricular)

QRS-complex morphology (narrow: supraventricular origin; wide: supraventricular origin associated with bundle-branch block or ventricular origin)

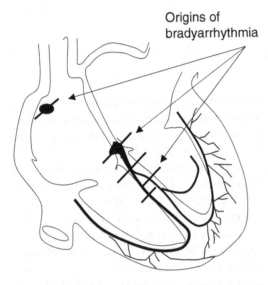

Origins of bradyarrhythmia

Fig. 4.1 Bradyarrhythmias can be the result of delayed/absent formation or conduction of the impulse at the level of the SA node, the AV node, the bundle of His, or the bundle branches

along the latter pathway is sufficiently slow, the stimulus reaches the blocked pathway after its refractory period is over, and it can thus be traversed in a retrograde fashion. Persistence of these electrophysiological conditions sets the stage for a self-sustaining arrhythmia.

The classic model of reentry is the Wolff-Parkinson-White syndrome (see Chap. 7), where the circuit consists of the normal conduction pathway through the AV node and an accessory pathway. Another example is AV nodal re-entry tachycardia. Here the circuit is the result of a second AV nodal pathway. Both of these conditions are related to *anatomical* reentry circuits (i.e., pre-existing pathways), but in other cases, the circuit is *functional*, that is, based solely on differences between contiguous fibers involving excitability, refractoriness, or both.

The third mechanism of tachyarrhythmia involves afterdepolarizations, oscillating currents present during the repolarization phase that are sometimes large enough in amplitude to generate repetitive firing. Under normal conditions, cardiac muscle fibers generate rhythmical electrical impulses as a manifestation of their spontaneous automaticity. In "triggered" activity, the action potential may be generated before phase 4 of the previous potential reaches the threshold level: afterdepolarizations therefore appear in relation to one or more of the previous electrical stimuli (which explains the term "triggered.") There are two types of afterdepolarizations (Fig. 4.4): those occurring before repolarization has been completed, during phase 2 or 3 of the action potential (early afterpotentials), and those that occur after repolarization has been completed, that is, in phase 4 (late afterdepolarizations). Early afterdepolarizations can be associated with the long-QT syndrome, hypokalemia, and therapy with antiarrhythmic drugs, such as quinidine, amiodarone, sotalol, and procainamide. Their appearance is facilitated by bradycardia, hypoxemia, and acidosis. A typical characteristic

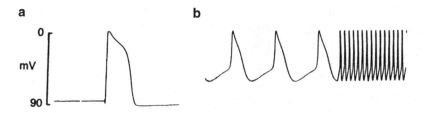

Fig. 4.2 Action potential of a cardiomyocyte under normal (**a**) and abnormal (**b**) conditions. In (**b**), the increased slope of phase 4 of the potential facilitates the onset of an arrhythmia

The mechanism of reentry

Extrasystole

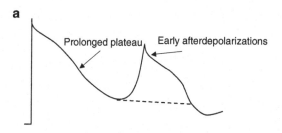

Fig. 4.3 Schematic representation of a re-entry circuit. *Left*: Under normal conditions, the impulse is simultaneously transmitted along the two conduction pathways. *Center*: In the presence of extrasystole and two pathways that differ in conduction velocity and refractoriness, the ectopic impulse moves ahead along the slow pathway (A), which is already excitable. Anterograde transmission along the fast pathway (B), which is still refractory, is blocked. *Right*: When the fast pathway becomes excitable again, the wavefront travels along it in a retrograde direction, perpetuating the reentry circuit

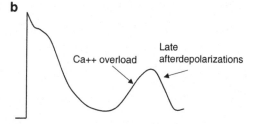

Fig. 4.4 Afterdepolarizations. (**a**) An early afterdepolarization occurs during phase 3 of the transmembrane action potential, which exhibits a prolonged plateau phase. (**b**) Late afterdepolarizations occur at the end of phase 4, when the potential has almost reached its resting value

of this phenomenon is a sequence of long-short R-R cycles right before onset of the arrhythmia (Fig. 4.5): reducing the length of the R-R cycle increases the duration of the action potential, as reflected by prolongation of the QT interval, and renders repolarization less homogeneous, a situation that can trigger repetitive ventricular responses. Late afterdepolarizations are typically associated with digitalis toxicity and with elevated catecholamine or calcium levels.

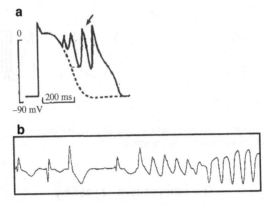

Fig. 4.5 Torsades de pointes triggered by early afterdepolarizations. The third complex represents a ventricular extrasystole followed by a long pause. The fourth complex is morphologically similar to the basal complex, but its QT interval is prolonged, and it is followed by a ventricular extrasystole that triggers the torsades de pointes. This extrasystole "closes" an RR cycle that is shorter than its predecessor (long-short sequence)

The Bradyarrhythmias

5

Introduction

The excitation-conduction system of the heart is controlled by the sinoatrial (SA) node, which is located in the right atrium, near the junction between the atrium and the superior vena cava. The SA node emits rhythmic electrical impulses at a higher rate than the rest of the cardiac tissue, including the atrioventricular (AV) node, which fires at rates ranging from 40 to 60 beats per minute (bpm), and other segments of the conduction system and the myocardial tissue itself (20–40 bpm) (Fig. 5.1). As noted early, *arrhythmias* are anomalous cardiac rhythms caused by the abnormal formation and/or conduction of the electrical impulse. They can be broadly classified as *tachyarrhythmias*, characterized by rapid heart rates exceeding 100 bpm, and *bradyarrhythmias*, with slow rates of less than 60 bpm.

Useful insight into the bradyarrhythmias can be obtained with intracardiac ECG, which is performed with a catheter electrode placed inside the cardiac chambers. The tracing obtained with this technique (Fig. 5.2) includes three main polyphasic elements:

- the A deflection, which represents activation of the atria;
- the H deflection, which corresponds to activation of the common trunk of the His bundle and has a normal duration of approximately 20–25 ms;
- the V deflection, which reflects activation of the ventricular myocardium.

If the surface and intracardiac ECGs are recorded simultaneously, three important intervals can be measured:

- The PA interval, which is measured from the onset of the P wave on the surface ECG to the first rapid A deflection. It represents the time required for the stimulus to travel from the SA node to the AV node (normally 15–25 ms).
- The AH interval, which is measured from the onset of the A deflection to the onset of the H deflection. It reflects the conduction time through the AV node (normally 60–120 ms).
- The HV interval, from the onset of the H deflection to the first rapid component of the V deflection, represents the time needed for depolarization of the His bundle, the bundle branches, and the Purkinje network (normally 35–55 ms).

These elements are necessary for subsequent understanding of the locations of atrioventricular blocks (AVBs) and their clinical significance and prognostic implications.

M. Romanò, *Text Atlas of Practical Electrocardiography*,
DOI 10.1007/978-88-470-5741-8_5, © Springer-Verlag Italia 2015

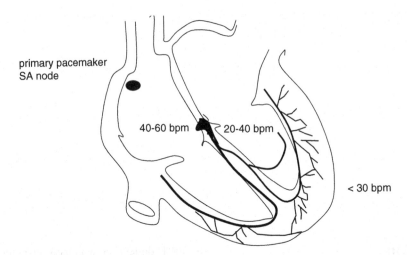

Fig. 5.1 The cardiac conduction system. The SA node is located in at the junction between the right atrium and the superior vena cava. The AV node is located in the right atrium near the coronary sinus. The bundle of His is located at the septal level. It divides to form the right and left bundle branches, which supply the right and left ventricles, respectively. The left bundle branch divides to form the anterosuperior and posteroinferior fascicles

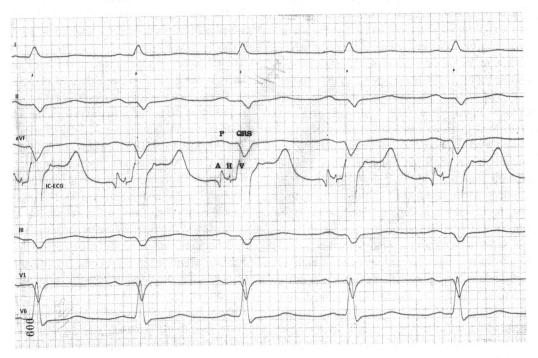

Fig. 5.2 Comparison of surface ECG tracings (leads I, II, III, aVF, V1, and V6) and intracardiac ECG (IC-ECG) tracing (4th from the top). The three main elements of the IC-ECG are seen: the **A** deflection (representing activation of the atrium); the **H** deflection (activation of the His bundle); and the **V** deflection (activation of the ventricular myocardium). See text for details on measurement of the PA, AH, and HV intervals. Paper speed: 100 mm/sec

D_1 ------------------ I
D_2 ------------------ II
D_3 ------------------ III
aVF --------------- aVF
V1 ------------------ V1
V6 ------------------ V6
Endo ---------------- IC-ECG

Table 5.1 Italian association of hospital cardiologists classification of the arrhythmias (from Alboni et al., 1999)

Tachycardias			
Supraventricular	Ventricular	Bradycardias	Premature beats
Sinus tachycardia	Ventricular tachycardia (VT)	Sinus bradycardia	Supraventricular premature beats
Atrial tachycardia	– nonsustained VT	Sinus arrhythmia	Ventricular premature beats
Atrial flutter (AFL)	– sustained monomorphic VT	Sinoatrial blocks	
– typical	– fascicular VT	Sinus arrest	
– atypical	– outflow-tract VT	AV blocks (AVBs)	
Atrial fibrillation (AF)	– polymorphous VT	– first degree	
– Paroxysmal	– Torsade de pointes	– second degree	
– Persistent	Ventricular fibrillation	• Wenckebach	
	Accelerated idioventricular rhythm (AIVR)	• Mobitz 2	
– Permanent		• 2:1	
		• Advanced	
		– third degree	
		AV dissociation	
AV nodal reentrant tachycardia (AVNRT)			
– slow-fast			
– fast-slow			
– slow-slow			
Atrioventricular reentrant tachycardia (AVRT) caused by:			
– an orthodromic manifest (WPW) accessory pathway			
– an antidromic manifest (WPW) accessory pathway			
– a concealed accessory pathway			
– a concealed, slow-conduction accessory pathway (Coumel type)			
– nodoventricular or nodofascicular fibers (Mahaim type)			
Junctional ectopic tachycardia			

Classification and Electrocardiographic Characteristics

Several arrhythmia classification systems have been proposed at the Italian and international levels. Here, we will use the system proposed some years ago by the Italian Association of Hospital Cardiologists (Table 5.1).

Arrhythmias Caused by Abnormal Impulse Formation

Healthy individuals at rest exhibit a sinus rhythm with rates ranging from 60 to 100 bpm. Variations can be caused by various factors related to the autonomic nervous system, the most common of which involves rate fluctuations related to the respiratory cycle (respiratory sinus arrhythmia).

Sinus Bradycardia

Sinus bradycardia is characterized by a regular rhythm and a rate of <60 bpm. It can be further classified as mild (rates between 50 and 59 bpm), moderate (40–49 bpm), or severe (<39 bpm) (Figs. 5.3 and 5.4). It is important to recall that in young, healthy subjects, nocturnal sinus rhythms at rates of 35–40 bpm are considered normal.

Fig. 5.3 Mild sinus bradycardia (approx. rate: 55 bpm)

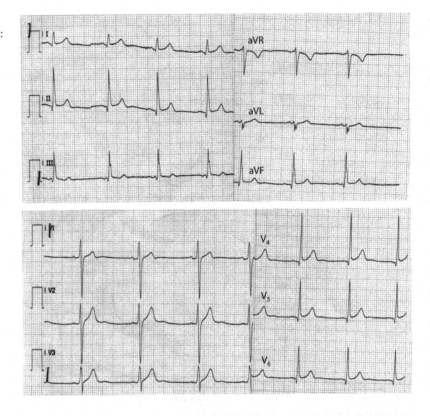

Fig. 5.4 Severe sinus bradycardia (approx. rate: 27 bpm)

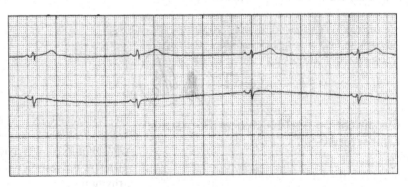

Sinoatrial Blocks and Sinus Arrest

These arrhythmias are caused by abnormal impulse formation or propagation from the SA node to the atrial myocardium, and they generally occur in an intermittent fashion. The most common type of sinoatrial block is a second-degree 2:1 block. It is characterized on ECG by a pause lasting twice as long as the preceding P-P cycle, during which no P waves are seen (Fig. 5.5). In contrast, sinus arrest involves a period of asystole that is more than twice as long as the baseline P-P cycle (Fig. 5.6). Junctional or ventricular escape beats may appear after sinus pauses of variable duration (Figs. 5.7 and 5.8).

Fig. 5.5 Second-degree 2:1 sinotrial block. The P-P cycle preceding the block (which occurs after the second complex from the left) has a duration of 1080 ms, half as long as the 2220-sec P-P cycle that includes the pause

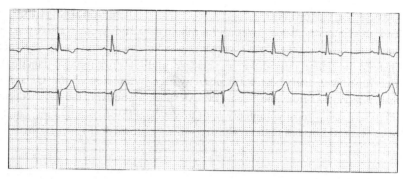

Fig. 5.6 Sinus arrest with an asystolic pause lasting approximately 2800 ms during which no electrical activity is recorded

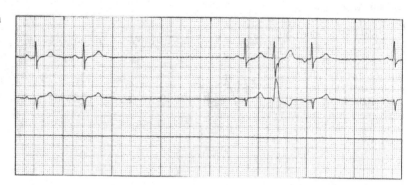

Fig. 5.7 Junctional escape (fourth complex) following sinus arrest. The junctional origin of the rhythm is reflected by the QRS morphology, which is similar to that seen during the sinus rhythm

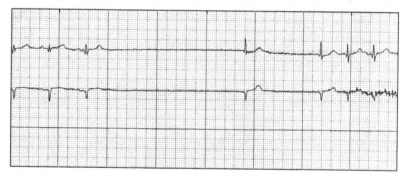

Fig. 5.8 Severe sinus bradycardia with ventricular escape beats (second and fourth complexes) and fusion beats (third complex) with morphology midway between those of the normal QRS and the ventricular complex

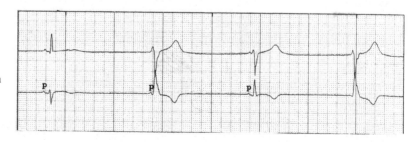

Wandering Pacemaker

This arrhythmia is characterized by morphologic variations involving the P wave, with progressive changes in polarity (positive to negative and vice-versa) with every beat. It is caused by pacemaker migration from the SA to the AV node (Fig. 5.9) and is most commonly seen in young persons, at rest or during the night.

Junctional Rhythm

If SA node activity is depressed, the stimulus may arise in the AV node (also known as the atrioventricular junction). The morphology and duration of the QRS complex in this case are similar to those seen during normal sinus rhythm. P waves, when present, are negative in the inferior leads and positive in lead aVR (Fig. 5.10)

Fig. 5.9 Wandering pacemaker manifested by morphological variations in the P waves, consisting in progressive beat-by-beat changes in polarity, from positive (reflecting the sinus origin) to negative (junctional origin), and shortening of the PR interval

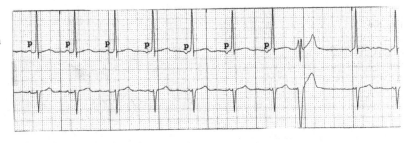

Fig. 5.10 Junctional rhythm. The P wave is negative in the inferior leads and positive in aVR, reflecting retrograde atrial activation that spreads upward and toward the right. Note that the PR interval is <120 sec

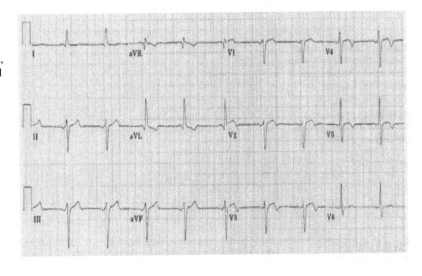

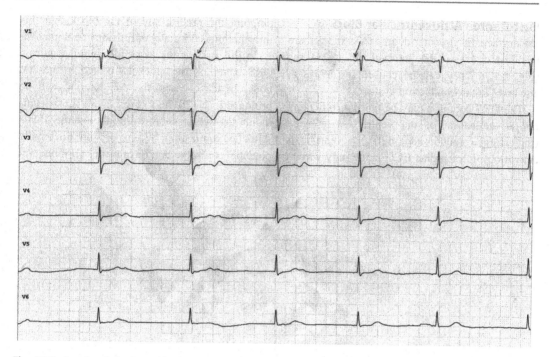

Fig. 5.11 Junctional rhythm with a rate of 30 bpm. The sinus and junctional activities are dissociated: P waves (*arrows*) are visible in the terminal portions of the first and second QRS complexes and then re-appear before the QRS

with a PR interval of <120 ms; they may also be absent and are sometimes obscured by the QRS complex (Fig. 5.11).

Conduction Disorders

These disorders include various types of ECG alterations, alone or in combination, caused by delayed or blocked transmission of the electrical stimulus at some point in the conduction system. Identifying the specific location of an AV block is fundamental for defining the prognosis and the indication for permanent cardiac pacing. These blocks are thus classified as supra-Hisian (delay located in the AV node), intra-Hisian (block in the His bundle), or infra-Hisian (block at the level of the bundle branches). The latter two have the least favorable prognoses, and higher-grade blocks of these types are indisputable indications for implantation of a permanent pacemaker.

Intracardiac ECG can reliably locate the site of an AV block. However, there are also specific surface ECG criteria that can be used to guide the diagnosis. In general, a narrow QRS complex (<120 ms) is indicative of a supra-Hisian block (especially first- or second-degree Mobitz type 1 or complete blocks). Regardless of the QRS morphology, AV node involvement should be suspected when blocks of increasing degrees are seen in the same tracing (first-degree block to second-degree Wenckebach-type block and on to higher degrees.)

First-Degree Atrioventricular Block

On surface ECGs, first-degree AV blocks are manifested by a PR interval of >200 ms (Fig. 5.12). They can be caused by delays at any level in the conduction system.

The QRS complex may be narrow (reflecting normal activation of the ventricles) or wide (indicating a concomitant delay in ventricular activation). Intracardiac ECG is the only way to pinpoint the precise site of the block, but this information is normally of little practical interest.

In 90 % of cases associated with a narrow QRS complex, the block is located in the AV node. In these cases, the AH interval will be prolonged (>120 ms) (Fig. 5.13). Less commonly the delay occurs within the bundle of His (H deflection lasting >25 ms or split His bundle potential) or in the bundle branches (HV interval

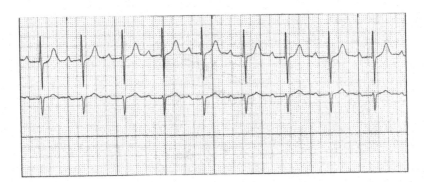

Fig. 5.12 First degree AVB with a PR interval of approximately 300 ms. The duration of the QRS complex is normal, so the block is located in the AV node

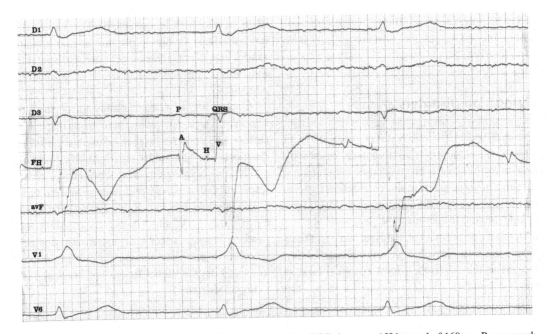

Fig. 5.13 First-degree AVB located in the AV node. Intracardiac ECG shows an AH interval of 160 ms. Paper speed: 100 mm/sec

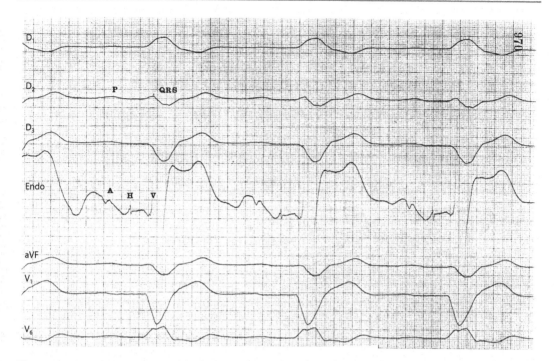

Fig. 5.14 First-degree AVB located in the bundle branches (HV interval of 90 ms), with an AH interval near the upper normal limits (115 ms) and a QRS complex with left bundle-branch-block morphology. Intracardiac recording, paper speed: 100 mm/sec

of >55 ms). AV node involvement may also be the cause of first-degree AV blocks associated with bundle branch blocks, but intra- or infra-Hisian blocks are more common than in cases characterized by a narrow QRS complex (Fig. 5.14).

Second-Degree Atrioventricular Block

There are several types.

Second-degree Mobitz type 1 (or Wenckebach-type) AV block. This intermittent disorder of conduction is characterized by a PR interval that increases progressively, beat-by-beat, until a P wave appears that is not followed by a QRS complex. Atrioventricular conduction then resumes, but the PR interval is shorter than it was prior to the appearance of the block (Fig. 5.15). Lengthening of the PR interval is typically greater in the first beats of the sequence, so there is a progressive reduction of the R-R cycle. In some forms, however, no fixed pattern

of PR interval prolongation can be discerned. In 70 % of cases, the block occurs in the AV node, and in these cases the QRS complex is almost always narrow. In the other 30 %, the presence of a bundle-branch-block pattern suggests possible involvement of the His-Purkinje system (the His bundle in 10 % of cases and the bundle branches in the remaining 15–20 %). Chronic AV blocks of this type are rare; paroxysmal blocks are more common, especially in young persons and athletes and during the night. Second-degree AV blocks originating in the AV node can be caused by drugs with negative dromotropic effects or by ischemic heart disease (typically acute inferior myocardial infarction) (Fig. 5.16).

Second-degree AV block, Mobitz type 2. In this case, there is a single nonconducted P wave, which is not preceded by any lengthening of the PR interval. It may occur repeatedly with P-QRS ratios of 3:2 or 4:3 (Fig. 5.17). The QRS complex in these cases is almost always wide because the

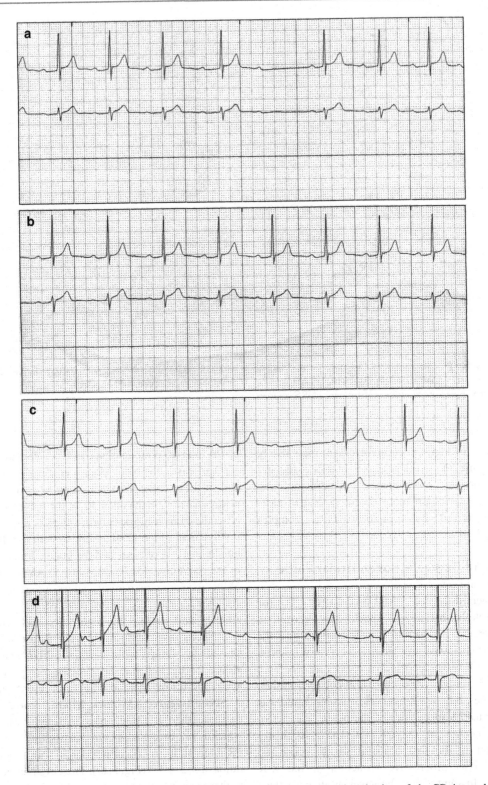

Fig. 5.15 (a–d) Second-degree AVB (Wenckebach type) with progressive lengthening of the PR interval that culminates in a nonconducted P wave. The QRS complex is normal in duration, so the block is located in the AV node

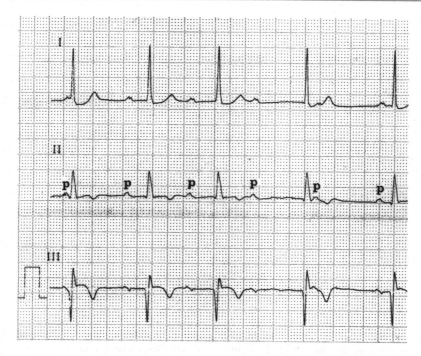

Fig. 5.16 Second-degree AVB (Mobitz 1) recorded during an acute inferior myocardial infarction. The location of the block is the AV node, and the QRS complex is narrow. ST segment elevation is present in the inferior leads

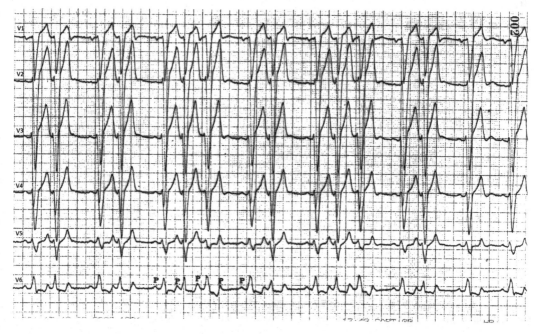

Fig. 5.17 Second-degree AVB (Mobitz 2), with a QRS complex indicative of LBBB. There is no appreciable variation in the duration of the PR interval during atrioventricular conduction

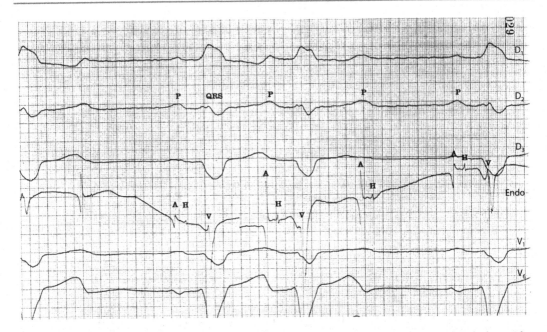

Fig. 5.18 Intracardiac recording obtained in the case shown in Fig. 5.17 reveals that the AV block is infra-Hisian. The nonconducted P wave seen in the surface leads corresponds to a block in atrioventricular conduction after the Hisian deflection, reflecting a conduction defect located in the bundle branches

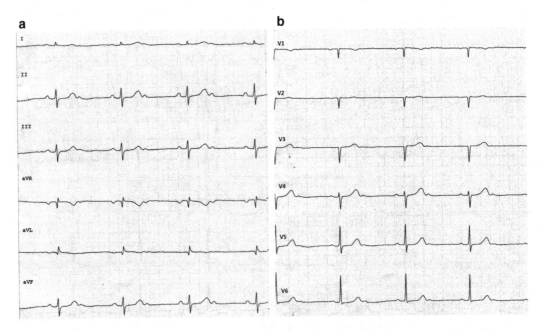

Fig. 5.19 (a–b) Second-degree 2:1 AVB located in the AV node and characterized by a narrow QRS complex

impulse is blocked in the His-Purkinje system (the His bundle in 35 % of cases, the bundle branches in 65 %) (Fig. 5.18).

Advanced second-degree AV block. This form is characterized by an AV ratio of 2:1 (Fig. 5.19), 3:1 (Fig. 5.20), or even higher

Fig. 5.20 (a–b) Severe bradycardia caused by a third-degree 3:1 AVB located in the AV node, as indicated by the narrow QRS complex. The *arrows* show P waves concealed within the ST segments

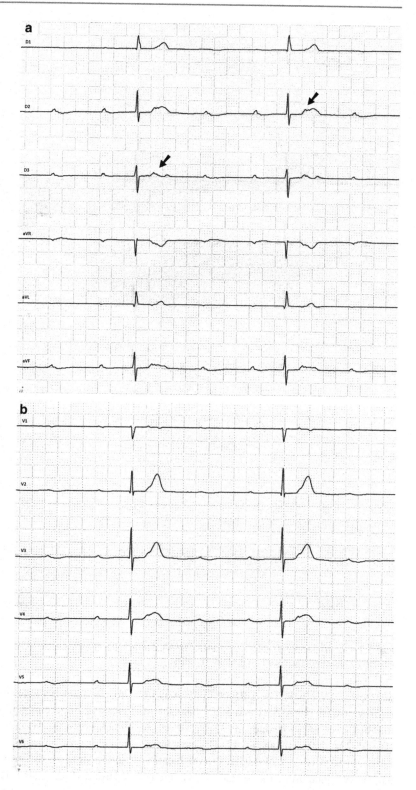

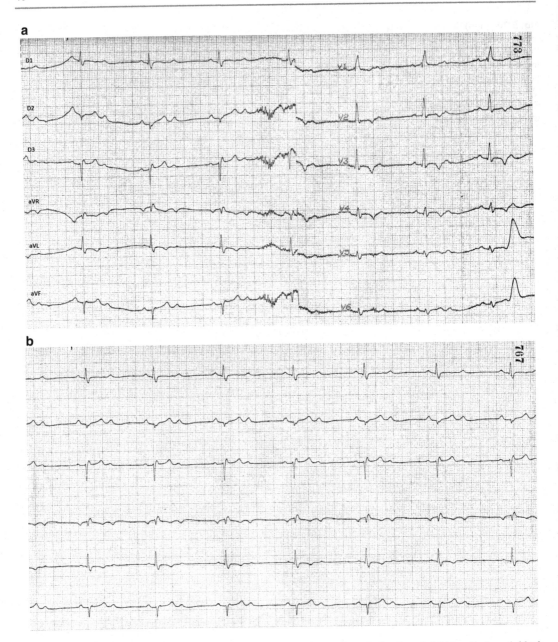

Fig. 5.21 (a–b) Second-degree 2:1 infra-Hisian AVB with QRS complexes indicative of right bundle-branch block (RBBB) and left anterior fascicular block (LAFB)

degrees of AV block. The QRS complex may be narrow or wide (Figs. 5.21 and 5.22). The site of the block is supra-Hisian in 33 % of cases (Fig. 5.23), intra-Hisian in 17 %, and infra-Hisian in 50 % (Fig. 5.24a). Clues to the location can be obtained from the surface ECG tracing when the AV conduction ratio is 1:1. AV node involvement is suggested by a narrow QRS, progressive lengthening of the PR interval before the block (as in the Wenckebach phenomenon), and reduction or regression of the block after the administration of atropine or during physical exertion (Fig. 5.24b). His-Purkinje involvement is more likely when bundle-branch-block

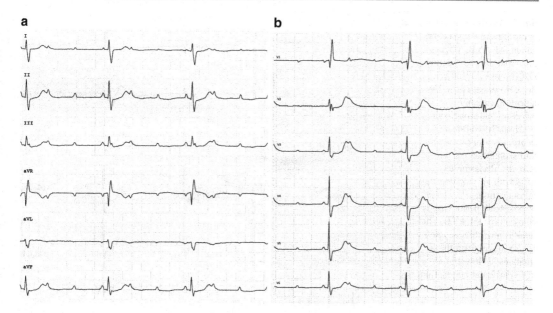

Fig. 5.22 (**a–b**) Second-degree 3:1 infra-Hisian AVB with widened QRS complexes indicative of complete RBBB and left posterior fascicular block (LPHB)

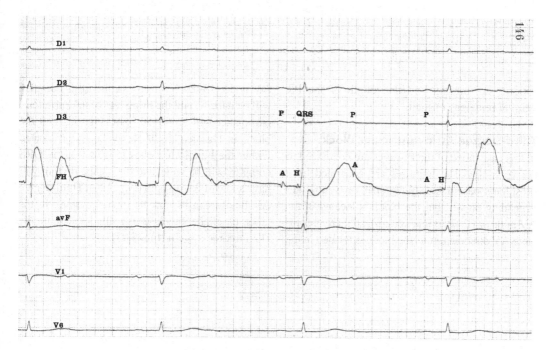

Fig. 5.23 Intracardiac ECG recording showing a 2:1 AVB with a narrow QRS complex, characterized by intermittent blockade of conduction in the AV node. The block occurs after the A deflection

Fig. 5.24 (a) Intracardiac recording showing second degree 2:1 AVB. Wide QRS complexes reflecting RBBB and LAFB. The block occurs after the H deflection (*arrow*), reflecting its infra-Hisian location. (**b**) Holter recording from a patient with second-degree narrow-QRS complex AVB with varying degrees of conduction. Wenckebach periodicity is followed by 3:1 AVB. The block is probably located in the AV node given the progressive slowing of atrioventricular conduction

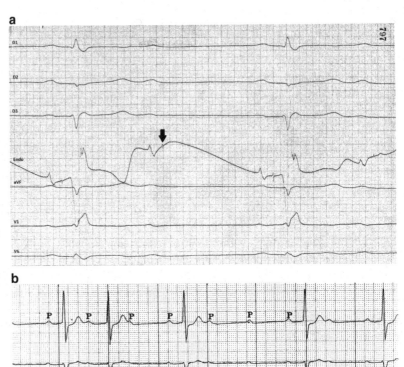

patterns are present and the length of the PR interval remains constant.

Third-Degree Atrioventricular Block

In this case, none of the P waves are conducted to the ventricles. The impulses are generated by a subsidiary pacemaker (junctional or ventricular depending on whether the block is located in the AV node or His-Purkinje system), so there is complete AV dissociation. If the block is located in the AV node (15–25 % of cases), the QRS complex will be narrow, and the firing rate of the subsidiary pacemaker will be 40–50 bpm (Fig. 5.25). If the block is Hisian (15–20 % of cases) or located within the bundle branches (55–70 %), the QRS complex will be wide, and the escape rhythm will have a rate of 25–40 bpm (Fig. 5.26). Third-degree AV blocks can be chronic or paroxysmal. In the latter case, the block is usually located in the His-Purkinje system (Fig. 5.27).

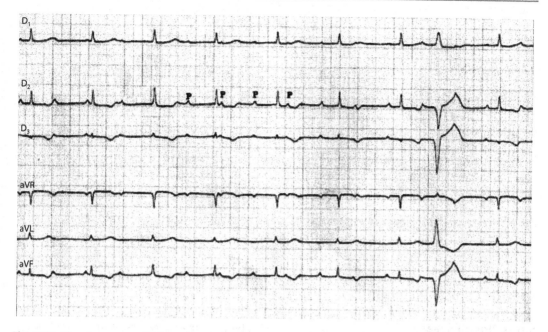

Fig. 5.25 Complete narrow-QRS-complex AV block located in the AV node: atrial activity is completely dissociated from that of the ventricles

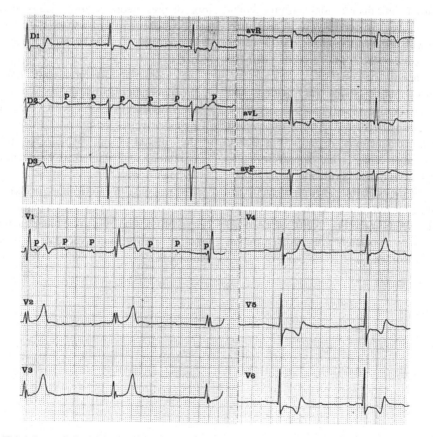

Fig. 5.26 Third-degree infra-Hisian AVB with ventricular escape rhythm with a rate of 32 bpm and RBBB+LAFB

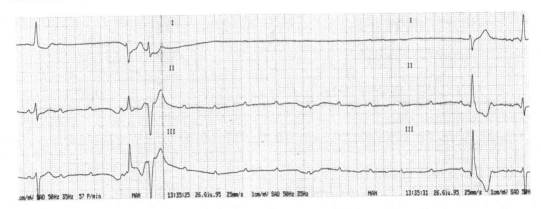

Fig. 5.27 Paroxysmal complete AVB with prolonged asystole (7200 ms) followed by ventricular escape

Specific Clinical Pictures

Sinus Node Disease

Also known as sinus node dysfunction and sick sinus syndrome, this disorder stems from cellular alterations in the SA node, which are often associated with degenerative changes in the atrial myocardium and/or the AV node. Its incidence in the general population is 0.06 %.

The ECG manifestations vary widely and include sinus bradycardia (Fig. 5.4), SA node blocks of varying degrees (Fig. 5.5), sinus arrest (Fig. 5.28), and junctional rhythms (Fig. 5.10), sometimes alternating with supraventricular tachyarrhythmias (atrial fibrillation, atrial flutter, and less commonly paroxysmal atrial tachycardia), a situation referred to as the bradycardia-tachycardia syndrome) (Fig. 5.29). Sinus node disease is often associated with atrioventricular conduction disorders.

The Carotid Sinus Syndrome

This syndrome is the result of hypersensitivity involving of baroreceptors of the carotid body, which regulate heart rate and arterial blood pressure. It causes recurrent episodes of syncope or presyncope. Carotid sinus hypersensitivity can be assessed and elicited by carotid sinus massage. It can be reproduced in three forms:

- the cardioinhibitory form, characterized by a predominantly bradyarrhythmic response;
- the vasodepressor form, with a predominantly hypotensive response;
- the mixed form, which is the most common and includes bradycardia and hypotension.

The response to carotid sinus massage is considered positive if it produces a pause of >3 sec (Fig. 5.30), a drop in systolic blood pressure of at least 50 mmHg, and syncopal or presyncopal symptoms.

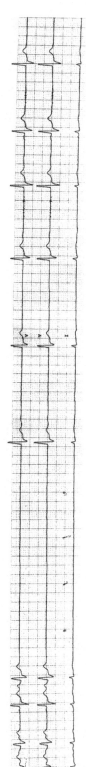

Fig. 5.28 Sinus arrest lasting 5120 ms is followed by a junctional escape rhythm. (The QRS complexes are not preceded by P waves and their duration is similar to that of the pre-arrest complexes: the origin of the escape rhythm is therefore located at the level of the atrioventricular junction.)

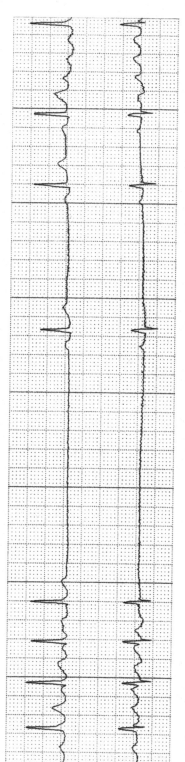

Fig. 5.29 Paroxysmal atrial flutter alternating with short bouts of sinus rhythm, which recurs after a pause of 2880 ms

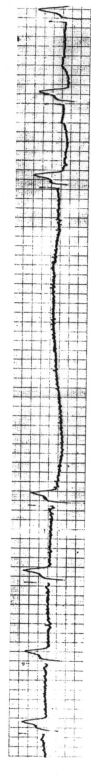

Fig. 5.30 Pathological response to a carotid sinus massage, which triggered asystole lasting 6680 ms

The Tachyarrhythmias

6

Introduction

The tachyarrhythmias comprise a variety of disorders ranging from isolated ectopic beats to repetitive arrhythmias arising in the atria or ventricles. See Chap. 5 (Table 5.1) for the classification of tachyarrhythmias proposed in 1999 by Alboni et al., which is still valid.

Ectopic Beats (Extrasystoles)

Extrasystoles are abnormal impulses originating at points in the myocardium other than the physiological pacemaker. Depending on the actual location, they are described as *supraventricular* or *ventricular*.

Supraventricular Ectopic Beats

These beats are characterized by a QRS complex that is premature (relative to the baseline R-R cycle) but, in general, morphologically similar to normal sinus complexes (Fig. 6.1). The complex may thus be narrow or, if there is an associated bundle-branch block (BBB), wide ectopic beats are referred to as *atrial* (if there is a P wave differing in morphology and axis from the sinus P wave and a PR interval of ≥ 120 ms) or *junctional* (when there is a negative P wave in the inferior leads and a PR interval of <120 ms or no atrial deflection at all). Supraventricular ectopic beats (SVEBs) can occur singly or in groups. They are generally followed by an incomplete or noncompensatory pause (i.e., one lasting less than twice as long as the normal P-P cycle), which is the result of SA node depolarization by the ectopic impulse. If the atrial extrasystole is very premature, it may reach the AV node while the latter is still refractory, and in this case it will not be conducted to the ventricles (nonconducted premature atrial complex or blocked atrial extrasystole). If instead the refractoriness is encountered in one of the bundle branches, the supraventricular impulse will be conducted with a QRS configuration unlike that of the baseline tracing, i.e., resembling that associated with bundle branch block (aberrantly conducted supraventricular extrasystole) (Fig. 6.2). SVEBs can also trigger short bursts of atrial tachycardia (Fig. 6.3).

M. Romanò, *Text Atlas of Practical Electrocardiography*,
DOI 10.1007/978-88-470-5741-8_6, © Springer-Verlag Italia 2015

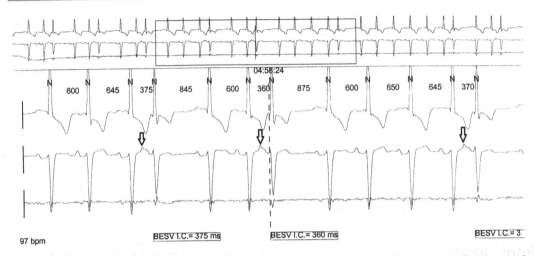

Fig. 6.1 Atrial extrasystoles documented by Holter recording. Compared with the baseline rhythm, the fourth, seventh, and last QRS complexes are premature but morphologically normal, and each is preceded by a P wave (*arrows*)

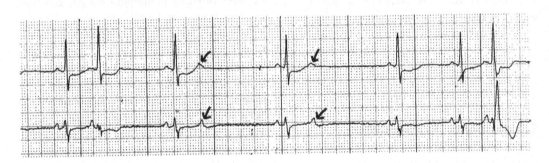

Fig. 6.2 Holter recording showing repetitive atrial extrasystoles. The second complex is conducted with partial aberrancy (QRS slightly different from baseline complexes). The third and fourth QRS complexes are followed by a premature P wave that is not conducted (nonconducted premature atrial complex or blocked atrial extrasystole). The result is severe bradycardia that can easily be misinterpreted. The key to the correct diagnosis is the lower tracing, which shows distortion of the T wave by the nonconducted premature P wave (*arrows*). The last complex is an atrial extrasystole that has been aberrantly conducted (right bundle-branch-block pattern)

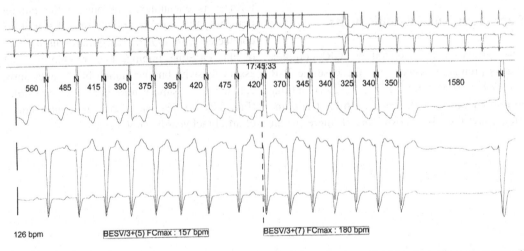

Fig. 6.3 During normal sinus rhythm, an atrial extrasystole can trigger a short run of atrial tachycardia, as documented by this Holter recording

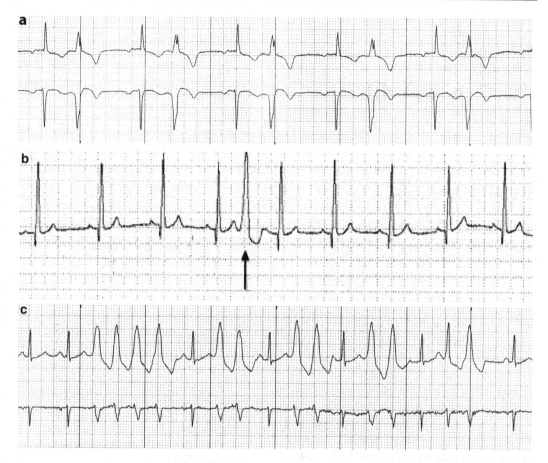

Fig. 6.4 Ventricular extrasystoles. (**a**) Bigeminy. The morphology of the premature QRS complexes is different from that of the normal complexes, and they are not preceded by atrial waves. There is also a compensatory pause, whereas in (**b**) the extrasystole is not followed by a compensatory pause and is therefore referred to as interpolated extrasystole. In this case, the phenomenon produces only a slight increase in the normal QRS cycle secondary to mildly delayed of conduction of the sinus impulse to the ventricles (PR interval longer than that of the baseline rhythm). (**c**) The morphology of the third complex from the right is midway between that of a normally conducted and ectopic QRS complexes. See text for details

Ventricular Ectopic Beats

If the premature complex is morphologically different from that of the baseline tracing (i.e., wide QRS complex) and not preceded by an atrial wave, the extrasystole is ventricular in origin. These ventricular ectopic beats (VEBs) may occur in isolated form, in bigeminal or trigeminal patterns (characterized by a VEB after every one or two sinus beats, respectively) (Fig. 6.4a), or in couplets or triplets. (The rapid succession of three or more VEBs with a rate >100 bpm is usually referred to as unsustained ventricular tachycardia [VT].) VEBs are followed by a compensatory pause (i.e., one that is twice as long as the previous R-R cycle) (Fig. 6.4a), because in

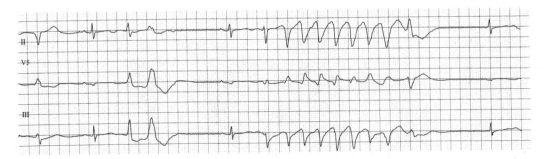

Fig. 6.5 Heart monitor recording showing obvious prolongation of the QT interval and premature ventricular extrasystoles capable of triggering episodes of VT

most cases the extrasystole does not depolarize the SA node, and the latter continues to emit impulses at its own discharge rate. Sometimes, however, the VEB fails to retrogradely penetrate the AV node or penetration is incomplete: in these cases the postextrasystolic sinus impulse will be conducted to the ventricles with a slight delay, as compared with normal atrioventricular conduction (Fig. 6.4b). When the rates of the normal and ectopic QRS complexes are similar, the morphology of the complexes may be intermediate between that observed during a normally conducted rhythm and that of the ectopic beat (fusion complex) (Fig. 6.4c). Particular attention should be reserved for premature VEBs falling near the peak of the previous T wave (the R-on-T phenomenon), which can provoke protracted tachyarrhythmic events, especially in the presence of repolarization abnormalities, such as QT interval prolongation (Fig. 6.5).

Table 6.1 Classification of the supraventricular tachyarrhythmias

Sinus tachycardia
Atrial tachycardia
Atrial flutter
– typical
– atypical
Atrial fibrillation
Atrioventricular nodal reentrant tachycardia (AVNRT)
– slow-fast
– fast-slow
Atrioventricular reentrant tachycardia (AVRT)
– caused by a manifest (WPW) accessory pathway. Orthodromic AVRT
– caused by a manifest (WPW) accessory pathway. Antidromic AVRT
– caused by a concealed accessory pathway
– caused by concealed, slow-conduction accessory pathway (Coumel-type)
– caused by nodoventricular or nodofascicular fibers (Mahaim-type)
Wolff-Parkinson-White syndrome (WPW)

The Supraventricular Tachyarrhythmias

This group includes numerous arrhythmias originating in the atria or the AV node (Table 6.1).

Sinus Tachycardia

Sinus tachycardia is characterized by a heart rate exceeding 100 bpm and P-waves that are normal in both morphology and axis (Fig. 6.6).

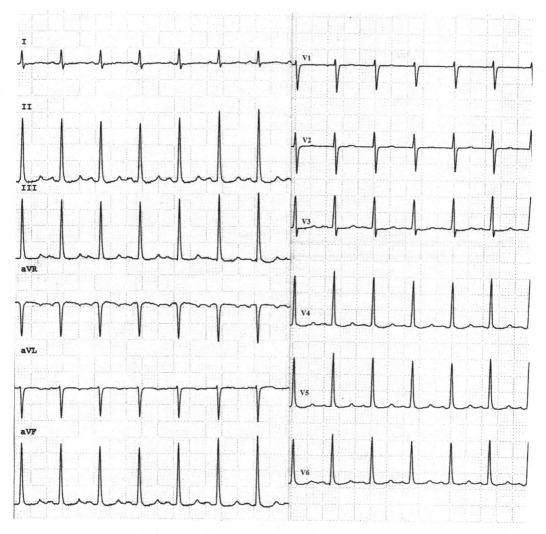

Fig. 6.6 Sinus tachycardia with a rate of approximately 130 bpm. The P wave is morphologically normal with an axis of 60°, and the QRS complex is narrow

Atrial Tachycardia

This type of tachycardia is characterized by morphologically identical P waves, heart rates ranging from 150 to 250 bpm, and clearly discernible isoelectric lines between the atrial deflections. In most cases, conduction of the atrial impulses to the ventricles is blocked. The AV ratio is usually 2:1 (although 1:1 conduction is by no means rare, which complicates the surface ECG diagnosis), and a Wenckebach pattern is sometimes seen. This arrhythmia is generally the result of increased automaticity, which is manifested by the so-called warm-up phenomenon consisting of progressive rate increases soon after the onset of tachycardia and gradual slowing before it ends (Fig. 6.7). Morphological analysis can often localize the origin of the arrhythmia to the right or left atrium (Figs. 6.8, 6.9, and 6.10).

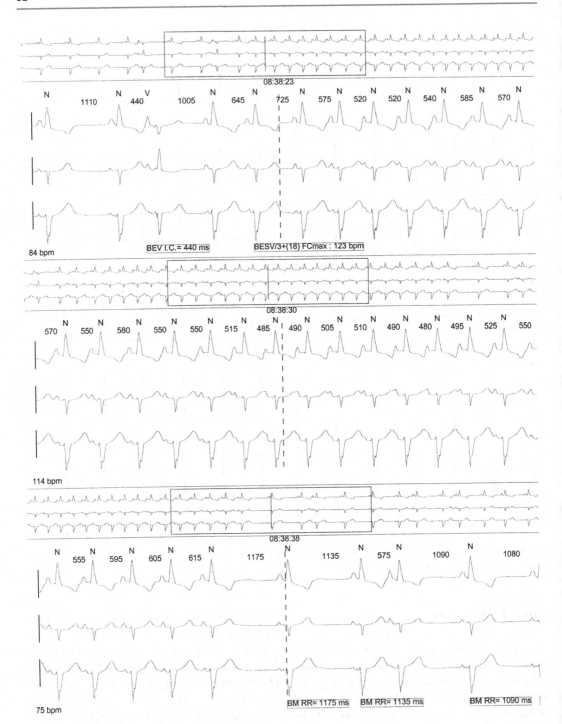

Fig. 6.7 Holter recording showing atrial tachycardia with progressive increases in the rate followed by progressive slowing prior to termination of the arrhythmia

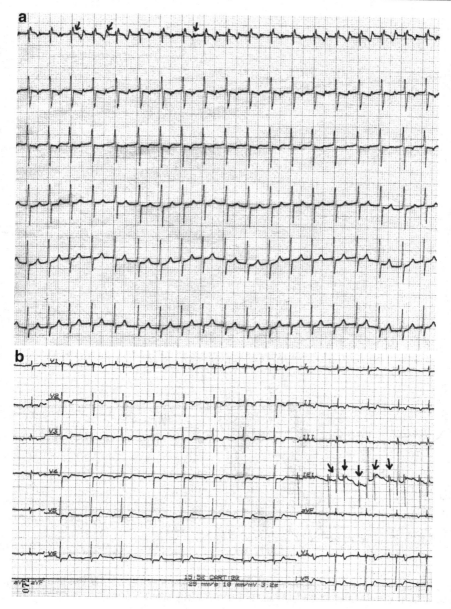

Fig. 6.8 ECG of a patient with supraventricular tachycardia (SVT). (**a**) Precordial lead tracings (top to bottom: V1 to V6). The QRS complexes are narrow. In lead V1 (top tracing) a P wave can be seen midway between two consecutive QRS complexes (*arrows*), and there is an r′ deflection that can be attributed to a second P wave. Diagnosis: atrial tachycardia with 2:1 conduction. (**b**) Intravenous administration of verapamil has reduced the ventricular rate, clearly revealing tachycardia with an AV conduction ratio of 2:1, as confirmed by the arrows in the esophageal tracing (fourth from the *top* on the *left*). The lead V1 tracing on the left (sixth from the *top*) shows QRS complexes characterized by a persistent r′ deflection and a P-P cycle identical to that seen before the verapamil was administered (**a**). The diagnosis is therefore atrial tachycardia with 2:1 conduction associated with incomplete RBBB. The origin of the atrial tachycardia is probably the right atrium (P-wave negativity in the inferior leads and positivity in V1)

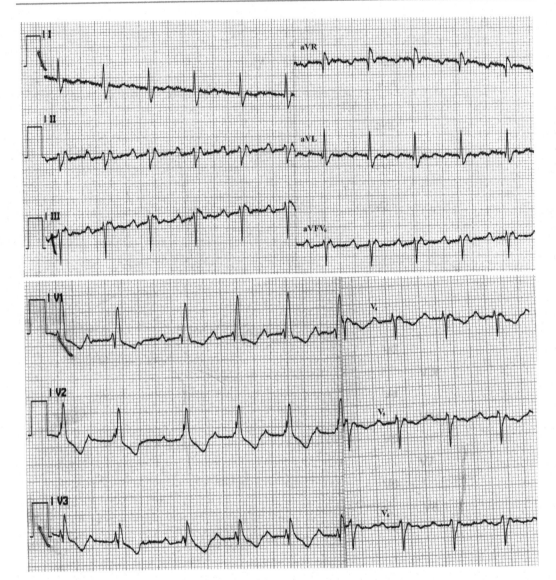

Fig. 6.9 Atrial tachycardia with 2:1 conduction that originates in the left atrium, as shown by P-wave positivity in all the precordial leads and the inferior limb leads and P-wave negativity in aVL and lead I

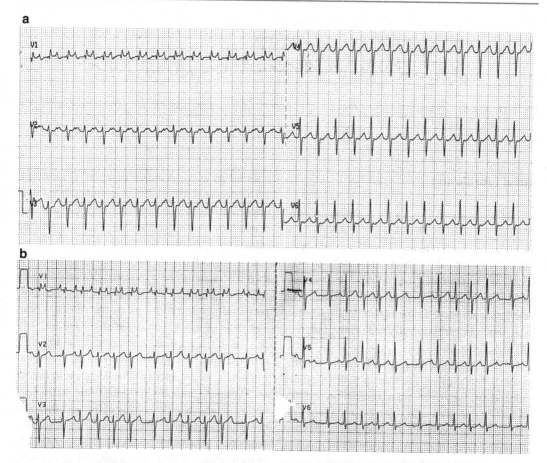

Fig. 6.10 (a) shows tracings from the precordial leads in a patient with narrow QRS complex tachycardia (rate 175 bpm), an obvious P wave after the QRS complex, and an atrioventricular conduction ratio of 1:1 (tachycardia with RP interval < PR′ interval). The diagnosis is by no means simple: is this a paroxysmal supraventricular tachycardia or atrial tachycardia? In (**b**) the response to vagal stimulation clarifies the situation, revealing a Wenckebach phenomenon without variations in the atrial cycle. The arrhythmia is therefore ectopic atrial tachycardia. A supraventricular reentry tachycardia would have been interrupted by the vagal maneuver. For details, see text on diagnosis of the supraventricular tachycardias

Multifocal Atrial Tachycardia

This supraventricular arrhythmia is characterized by an atrial frequency of >100 bpm and P waves with at least three different configurations (Fig. 6.11). The electrical basis is probably increased automaticity. It is commonly seen in patients with chronic respiratory disease.

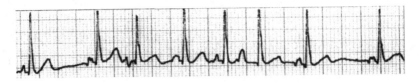

Fig. 6.11 This ECG contains three morphologically distinct P waves with different P-P, PR, and RR intervals, typical signs of multifocal atrial tachycardia

Atrial Fibrillation

Atrial fibrillation (AF) is a very common arrhythmia characterized by chaotic electrical activity in the atria with rates ranging from 350 to 600 bpm. Conduction of the atrial impulses to the ventricles is regulated and slowed by the AV node, which functions as a sort of filter. The ventricular response to the high-rate atrial activity is much lower, generally within the range of 100 to 150 bpm.

ECG diagnosis of AF is usually fairly straightforward. P waves as such are absent: they are replaced by rapid, irregular oscillations of the isoelectric line known as *f* waves, and the rhythmicity of the ventricular complexes is lost completely (Fig. 6.12). An exception to this rule is AF associated with an atrioventricular block (AVB) (Fig. 6.13): in this case the ventricular complexes occur regularly. As shown in Figs. 6.14 and 6.15, Holter monitoring may reveal phases in which the AVB is even more severe than that seen in Fig. 6.13.

On ECGs recorded during AF (and all other supraventricular arrhythmias as well), there may be morphologically aberrant ventricular complexes, reflecting intermittent or permanent bundle-branch block. When the aberrant complex is isolated and occurs after a short R-R interval preceded by a long R-R interval, it is referred to as an Ashman complex (Fig. 6.16). To understand the Ashman phenomenon, it is important to recall that for myocardial and conduction-system cells, the duration of the refractory periods (i.e., the interval during which the cells have not been repolarized and therefore cannot be re-excited by an external stimulus) generally decreases and increases proportionally with the length of the cardiac cycle. The cells of the AV node are an exception: they behave in the opposite manner and can thus fulfill their role as a filter in the presence of high-frequency atrial activity. The long cycle before an Ashman complex prolongs the refractory period of the bundle-branch cells, and the next complex is widened. The morphology is usually indicative of a block involving the *right* bundle branch, which normally remains refractory longer than the left bundle branch. When the associated bundle-branch block is permanent, the diagnosis is generally simple (Figs. 6.17, 6.18, and 6.19).

In rare cases, the *f* waves cannot be clearly visualized on surface tracings: in these cases the differential diagnosis must include atrial standstill, which is characterized by the absence of electrical and mechanical activity in the atria. In some cases, the defect reflects the progression of atrial disease, in others the expression of a genetically determined rhythm disorder (Fig. 6.20).

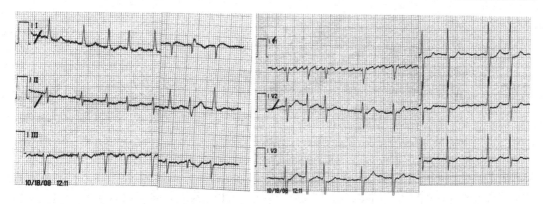

Fig. 6.12 ECG illustrating the peculiar characteristics of AF: absence of P waves, which have been replaced by fine oscillations of the isoelectric line known as *f* waves (rate 380/min), and completely irregular RR intervals

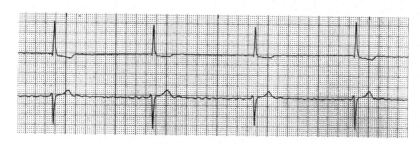

Fig. 6.13 AF associated with high-grade atrioventricular block (AVB) is slow and regular with a mean ventricular response rate of approximately 30 bpm

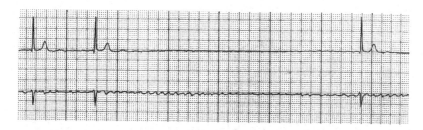

Fig. 6.14 AF characterized by a nocturnal asystolic pause lasting more than 5 seconds

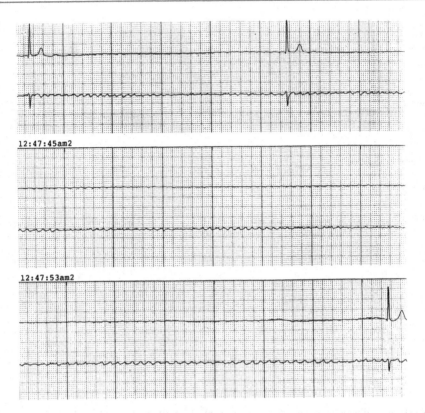

12:47:45am2

12:47:53am2

Fig. 6.15 Holter tracing documenting a period of asystole lasting more than 17 seconds and associated with syncope

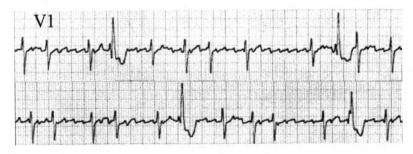

Fig. 6.16 The Ashman phenomenon. In this ECG tracing recorded in V1, the 4th and 10th QRS complexes of the upper strip and the 6th and 11th complexes of the lower strip have a complete RBBB morphology (rsR'). In this case, the origin of these complexes is supraventricular

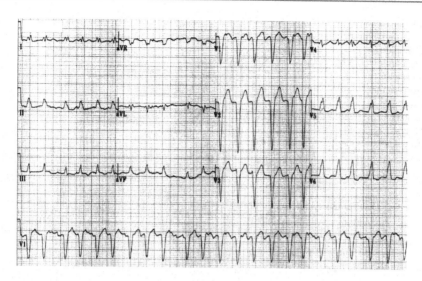

Fig. 6.17 Tachyarrhythmic AF in the presence of a left bundle-branch block (LBBB). The rhythm is irregular, and there are no discernible sinus P waves, but *f* waves are present, especially in V1. Typical associated LBBB

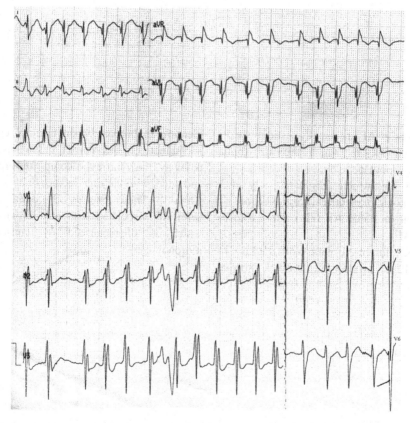

Fig. 6.18 Tachyarrhythmic AF with RBBB and Left posterior fascicular block. The QRS morphology in V1 is of the rsR′ type, a large S wave in V5 and V6, right axis deviation (+120°), and *f* waves in V1

Fig. 6.19 Atrial
fibrillation associated with
complete LBBB and
vertical electrical axis
(+120°). Evidence of
previous necrosis in the
mid-anterior wall (QS in
leads V1-3, I, and aVL),
f waves in V1,
numerous VEBs

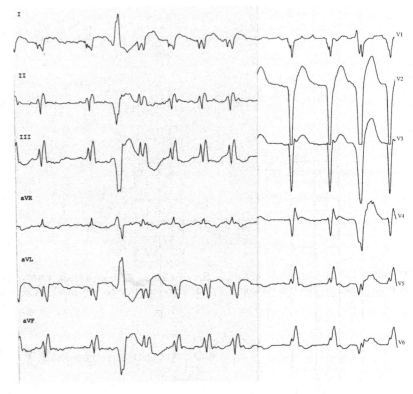

Three types of AF are usually distinguished:

1. paroxysmal AF in which the arrhythmia terminates spontaneously;
2. persistent AF, which terminates only after pharmacologic or electrical cardioversion;
3. permanent or stable AF (also referred to as chronic AF).

The association of AF with Wolff-Parkinson-White (WPW) syndrome deserves special mention. In this case, when the electrical impulse is conducted to the ventricles along an accessory pathway, the ventricular complexes are irregular and wide, with varying degrees of aberrancy (see Chap. 7). These features differentiate this form from AF associated with bundle-branch block, which is characterized by constant QRS morphology.

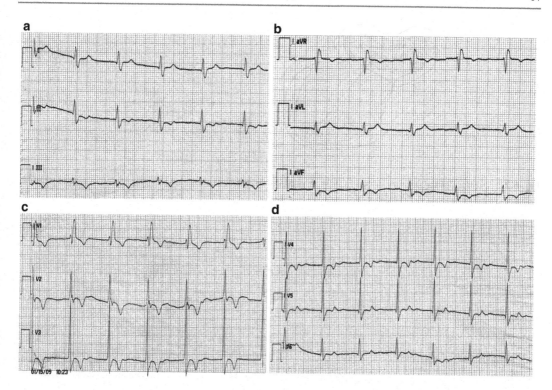

Fig. 6.20 This ECG is characterized by atrial standstill (the line between QRS complexes is essentially isoelectric, reflecting the absence of atrial electrical activity) and a regular junctional escape rhythm (rate 72 bpm) with RBBB conduction (**a–d**). The QRS complexes are unlikely to originate in the ventricles given their morphologies in leads V1 (rSR′), V6 (Rs), and I (RS)

Atrial Flutter

Atrial flutter (AFL) is a type of macro-reentrant atrial tachycardia (Fig. 6.21). Its electrocardiographic features include the absence of P waves and the presence of regular flutter waves (F waves) at rates of 250–350 bpm. As in AF, the AV-node "filter" limits the ventricular response, which rarely exceeds 150–160 bpm. The most common feature of the ECG is a 2:1 block of the impulses arriving from the atria (Figs. 6.22 and 6.23). In this case the nonconducted F wave may be concealed within the QRS complex or occur immediately after it. Poorly visualized F waves can be rendered manifest by interventions that slow atrioventricular conduction (carotid sinus massage, administration of verapamil, digitalis, or adenosine) (Fig. 6.24). There is typically no discernible isoelectric line between the F waves. In general, AFL can be easily diagnosed on a 12-lead surface ECG thanks to the presence

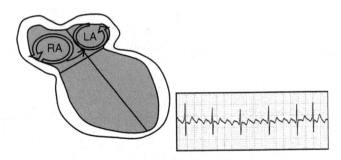

Fig. 6.21 Diagram of the re-entry circuit in typical atrial flutter: the activation wave is propagated in a caudocranial, counter-clockwise direction. *RA* right atrium, *LA* left atrium

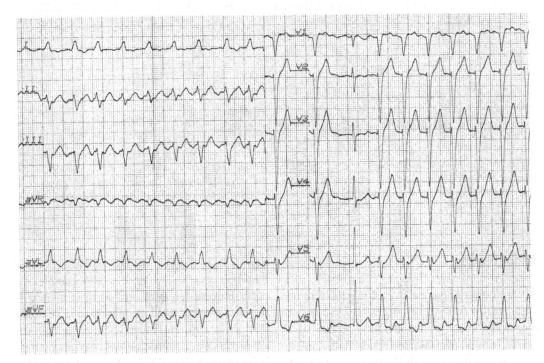

Fig. 6.22 Common CTI-dependent atrial flutter with 2:1 atrioventricular conduction. Saw-tooth F waves are negative in the inferior leads and positive in leads I, aVL, and V1, thus confirming the caudocranial progression of the atrial activation wave. See text for details

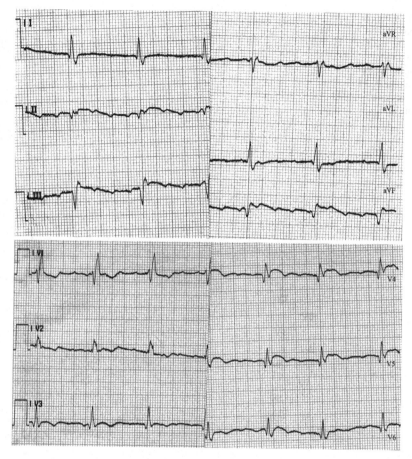

Fig. 6.23 Another case of counter-clockwise, CTI-dependent atrial flutter with F waves that are negative in the inferior leads and positive in V1. Associated complete RBBB and left anterior fascicular block (LAFB)

of F waves, which are most evident in the inferior leads and in V1.

There are different types of AFL. Data based on intracardiac recordings, particular those obtained during catheter ablation procedures, have increased our understanding of electrophysiological mechanisms. Various AFL classifications have been proposed: one of the most recent is shown in Table 6.2.

Classic atrial flutter is the result of a macro-reentrant circuit in the right atrium that involves the cavotricuspid isthmus (CTI) (CTI-dependent atrial flutter). The circuit is sustained by anatomical structures such as the *crista terminalis*, the Eustachian ridge, and the tricuspid annulus. In the "common" form of atrial flutter (which accounts for the majority of cases), the activation wave proceeds along the

Fig. 6.24 Narrow-QRS tachycardia shown to be atrial flutter on the basis of the response to a vagal maneuver: slowing of the ventricular rate revealed F waves in the precordial leads with a rate of 280 bpm

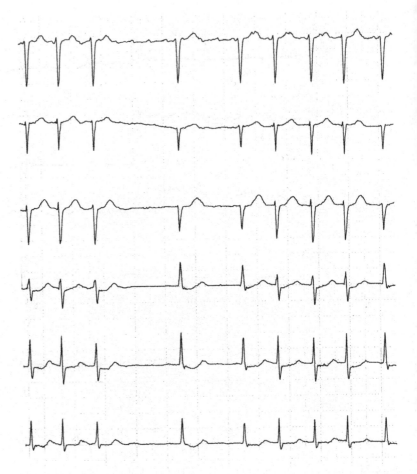

Table 6.2 Electrophysiological classification of atrial flutter[a]

1. CTI-dependent right atrial flutter.
   – Counterclockwise flutter (also known as common atrial flutter)
   – Clockwise flutter (also known as uncommon atrial flutter)
   – Double-wave reentry
   – Lower-loop reentry atrial flutter
   – Intraisthmus re-entry
2. Non-CTI-dependent right atrial flutter (atypical)
   – Scar-related atrial flutter
   – Upper-loop atrial flutter
3. Left atrial flutter
   1. Mitral annular flutter
   2. Scar- and pulmonary vein-related flutter
   3. Coronary-sinus flutter
   4. Left septal flutter

[a]Modified from Scheinman et al. Pacing Clin Electrophysiol 2004; 27:504-6

right aspect of the interatrial septum in a caudocranial direction, arrives at the roof of the right atrium and then descends along the free wall to the CTI in the lower part of the atrium (Fig. 6.21). Observed in the left anterior oblique projection, the stimulus moves through the circuit in a *counter-clockwise* direction. The ECG displays F waves that are negative in leads II, III, and aVF (with the typical saw-tooth configuration) and positive in V1, because in this case activation of the interatrial septum proceeds caudocranially and anteriorly (Figs. 6.22 and 6.23). In this case, the P wave, which is positive in V1, becomes progressively negative in the other precordial leads. In the "uncommon" form of atrial flutter, the F waves are positive in the inferior leads and negative in V1, reflecting spread of the activation wave in a *clockwise* manner (Fig. 6.25).

Fig. 6.25 Uncommon atrial flutter. The F waves are positive in the inferior leads and negative in V1, reflecting the craniocaudal, clockwise progression of atrial-activation

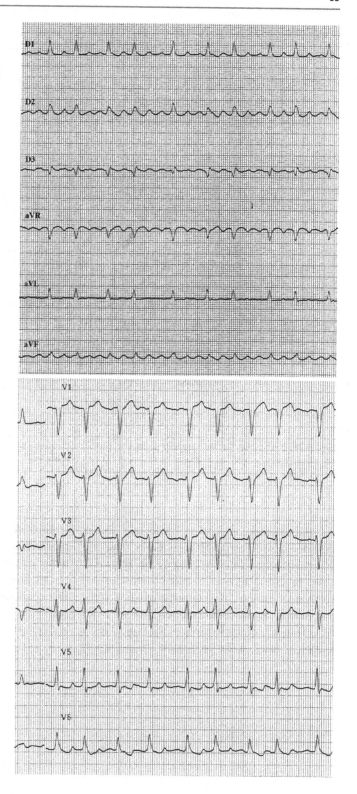

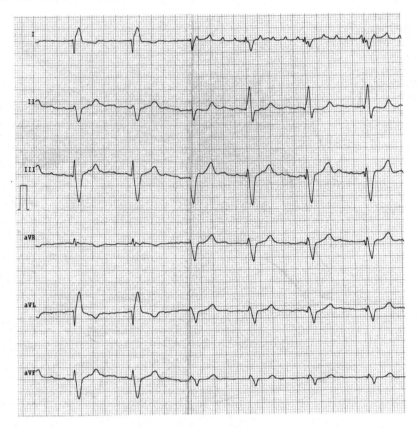

Fig. 6.26 Left atrial flutter originating in the mitral annulus in a patient with a prosthetic mitral valve. The F waves (approx. rate 300 bpm) are positive in V1 and positive but lower in voltage (<1 mV) in the inferior leads. A VVI pacemaker rhythm (see Chap. 10) is present

Isthmus-independent or atypical flutter includes a wide array of arrhythmias that are unrelated to the CTI. They are listed in Table 6.2. Their precise diagnosis is based almost exclusively on the results of electrophysiological studies. Indeed, atypical flutter often presents with ECG features similar to those of the typical form except in cases of flutter originating in the left atrium, where the amplitude of the F waves is reduced. The most common form of atypical flutter is related to a left-atrial macroreentrant circuit around the mitral annulus. The surface ECG in these cases reveals low-voltage F waves in the inferior leads and positivity in V1 and V2 (Figs. 6.26, 6.27, and 6.28).

Fig. 6.27 Atypical atrial flutter with 2:1 conduction originating in the left atrium: the F waves (rate 300 bpm) are positive in the inferior leads, negative with low voltage in the lateral leads (aVL and I), and positive in V1. The patient has a prosthetic mitral valve

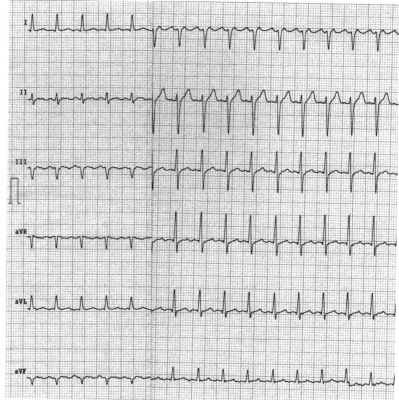

Fig. 6.28 Another case of left atrial flutter. The F-wave amplitude in the inferior leads is approximately 2 mV. The polarity is positive in the inferior leads and all the precordial leads and negative in the lateral leads (aVL and I)

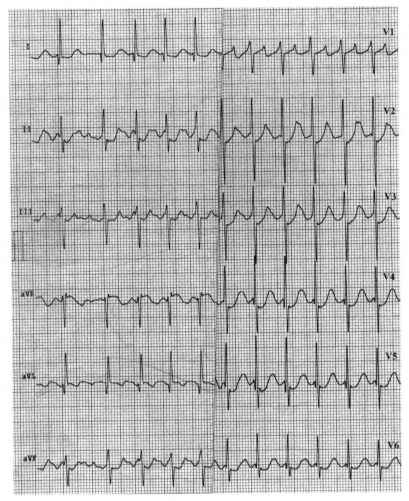

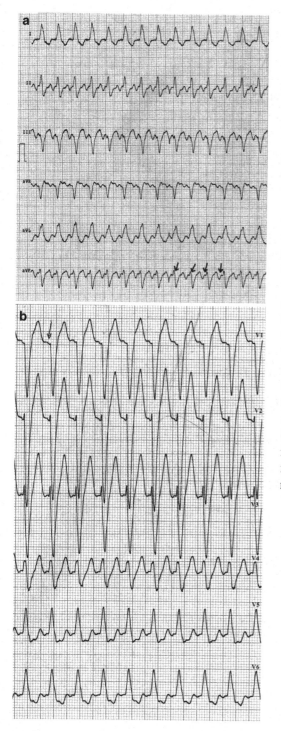

Like AF, atrial flutter can be associated with bundle-branch blocks: in this case the presence of F waves facilitates the diagnosis (Fig. 6.29). In very rare cases the flutter can be terminated with a vagal maneuver (Fig. 6.30). In recent years the increasing use of class IC antiarrhythmic drugs (e.g., flecainide, propafenone) to prevent AF has led to the appearance of a specific clinical and electrocardiographic entity known as *IC atrial flutter*. These sodium channel-blocking effects of these antiarrhythmics slow cardiac conduction, lengthening the F-F cycle and thereby converting AF into AFL. As the atrial rate decreases, the flutter waves may be conducted to the ventricles with a 1:1 ratio and an aberrant QRS configuration, which is caused by the high ventricular rate and the electrophysiological effects of the drugs on the bundle branches. The result is a broad-QRS-complex tachycardia, which is sometimes difficult to distinguish from VT (Fig. 6.31) and has hemodynamic effects that are just as poorly tolerated. An esophageal recording can be helpful in these cases: documentation of 1:1 atrioventricular conduction supports the suspicion of class IC flutter (Fig. 6.32). Transesophageal stimulation can interrupt the arrhythmia or transform it into atrial fibrillation, which in any case facilitates the diagnosis (Figs. 6.33 and 6.34).

Fig. 6.29 Common, typical atrial flutter with 2:1 AV conduction and associated with complete LBBB (**a**, **b**). Note that the F waves are negative in the inferior leads and positive in the precordials. The *arrows* highlight the 2:1 AV ratio

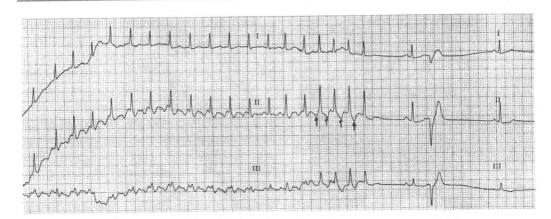

Fig. 6.30 Common, typical atrial flutter with 2:1 AV conduction (nonconducted F wave at the end of the QRS complex) and a cycle of 240 ms. During vagal stimulation, the duration of the flutter cycle increases from 280 ms (cycle delimited by the first *two arrows*) to 320 ms (between the second and third and the third and fourth complexes. The result of this minimal decrease in the atrial rate is a drop in the AV ratio from 2:1 to 1:1 and blocked conduction of the impulse along the flutter circuit

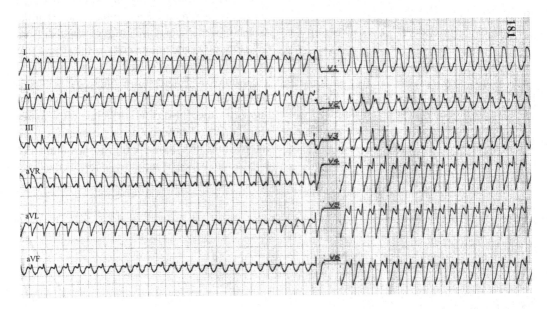

Fig. 6.31 IC atrial flutter with 1:1 atrioventricular conduction. The QRS morphology is aberrant with features suggestive of VT. Monophasic R waves are present in V1 and V2, an R/S ratio of < 1 in V6. Additional details on this case are shown in Figs. 6.32, 6.33, and 6.34

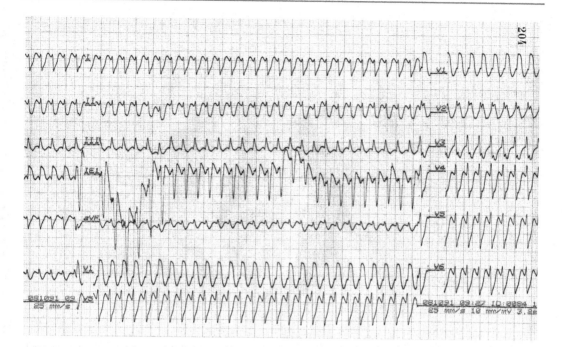

Fig. 6.32 Tracings from the case presented in Fig. 6.31. The fourth from the top is an esophageal recording that documents an AV ratio of 1:1, which supports a diagnosis of atrial arrhythmia with an AV ratio of 1:1 (see also Fig. 6.33)

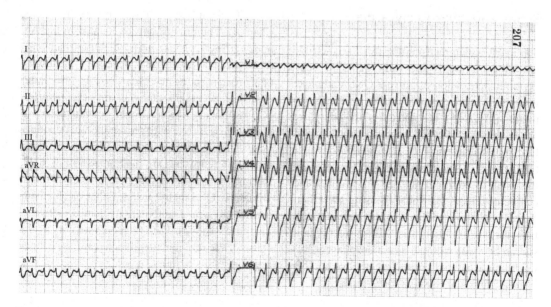

Fig. 6.33 Case presented in the previous two figures. Transesophageal stimulation reduces the QRS duration without altering the atrial and ventricular cycles, and an atrial wave appears at the end of the QRS in V1

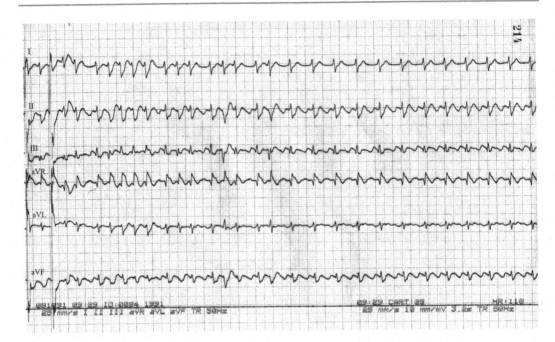

Fig. 6.34 Here the IC flutter with 1:1 conduction seen in Fig. 6.31 evolves toward classic atrial flutter with a predominant conduction ratio of 2:1. When the ratio drops to 1:1 (left-hand side of the tracing), the aberrant morphology of the QRS re-emerges

Supraventricular Tachycardia

Supraventricular tachycardia (SVT) is characterized by a rapid (generally 120–200 bpm), rhythmic succession of narrow QRS complexes resembling those recorded during a normal sinus rhythm (Fig. 6.35). In some cases, the complexes have a duration of >120 ms and a bundle-branch block (BBB) pattern (Figs. 6.36 and 6.37). Sometimes the BBB is preexisting; in other cases it is the result of the rapid rate. SVT with aberrancy can be distinguished from VT using the criteria described below in the section on ventricular tachycardias. If doubts arise, the correct diagnosis can be made with the aid of esophageal ECG recording, which will reveal whether or not there is atrioventricular dissociation.

SVT is usually caused by reentry (see Chap. 4). The circuit may be located in the AV node (atrioventricular nodal reentrant tachycardia) or include an accessory pathway (AV reciprocating tachycardia). In the latter case, the accessory pathway may be *manifest* (i.e., allowing bidirectional conduction) or *concealed* (i.e., one with retrograde-only conduction). The electrophysiological characteristics of these different types are diagrammed in Fig. 6.38. Reentry is responsible for approximately 90 % of all narrow QRS tachycardias. Other mechanisms include abnormal automaticity (sinus tachycardia, atrial tachycardia). Triggered activity is the cause of the rare junctional tachycardias secondary to digitalis toxicity.

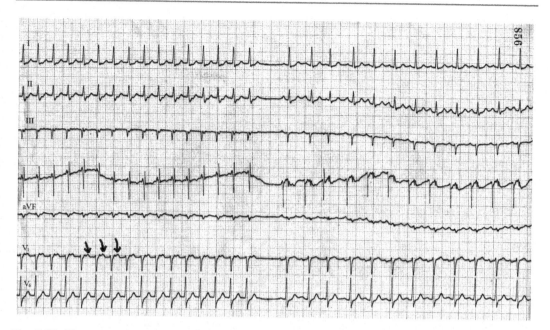

Fig. 6.35 Narrow-complex SVT interrupted by vagal maneuver. During the tachycardia, the QRS morphology resembles that seen during sinus rhythm. The fourth tracing from the top was recorded with an esophageal lead. It shows an AV ratio of 1:1 and a ventriculoatrial time of approximately 60 ms. Note the pseudo r′ in V1, suggestive of an AV nodal re-entry circuit (*arrows*)

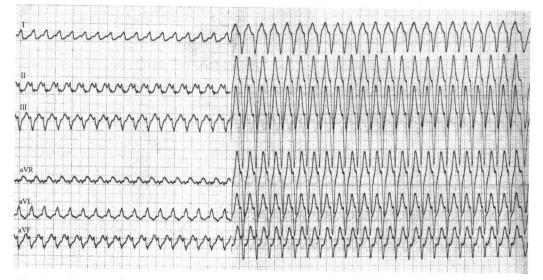

Fig. 6.36 AV node reentrant tachycardia conducted with an LBBB: the diagnosis is suggested by the absence of P waves and the typical LBBB morphology, which points to aberrancy rather than a ventricular origin of the arrhythmia. For details, see the section on Ventricular tachycardias

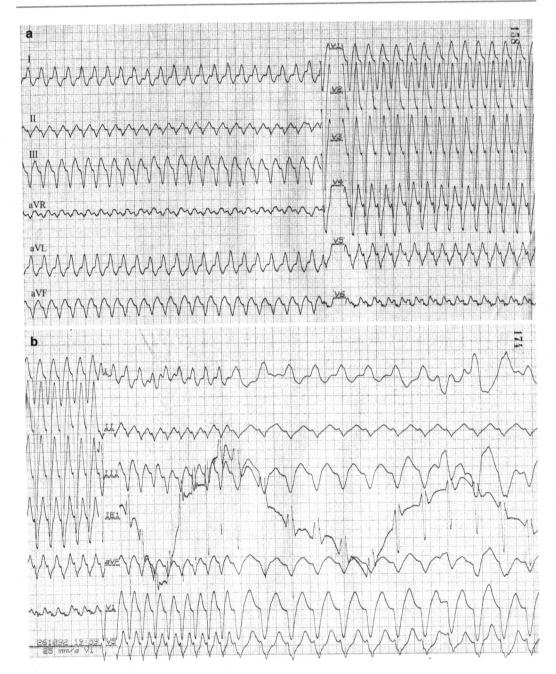

Fig. 6.37 SVT with aberrant conduction (complete LBBB with left axis deviation (**a**). In (**b**) the esophageal lead (fourth tracing from the *top*) shows a V-A interval of 40 ms, which localizes the origin of the SVT to the AV node. In the right half of the figure, the paper speed is 50 mm/sec

Two main types of supraventricular tachycardia can be distinguished on the basis of the relation between the P wave and the QRS complex that follows it: those characterized by a short RP interval and those with a long RP interval. The forms representing each type are shown in Table 6.3.

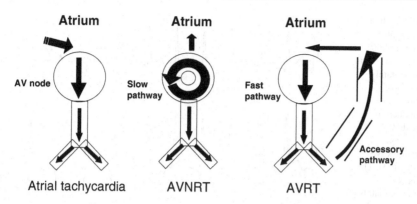

Fig. 6.38 *Left*: Diagram showing activation of the AV node, the His bundle, and the bundle branches during atrial tachycardia: the impulse originating in the atrium follows the normal conduction pathways. *Center*: Re-entry circuit associated with typical AV node reciprocating tachycardia: the impulse descends through the slow pathway (anterograde conduction) and returns toward the atria via the fast pathway (retrograde conduction). In this case the atria and the ventricles are activated almost simultaneously. *Right*: Re-entry circuit involving an accessory pathway (Kent bundle): anterograde transmission of the impulse occurs through the AV node, retrograde transmission through the accessory pathway. In this case atrial activation occurs after ventricular activation

Table 6.3 Types of narrow-QRS-complex tachycardias

Short RP interval (RP < PR) forms	Long RP interval (RP > PR) forms
AV node reentrant tachycardia	Sinus tachycardia
AV reentrant tachycardia	Sinus node reentrant tachycardia
Nonparoxysmal junctional tachycardia	Atrial tachycardia
	Permanent reciprocating junctional tachycardia (PJRT)
	Atypical AV reentrant tachycardia (fast-slow)

Short-RP Tachycardias

The short RP forms are by far the most frequent.

Atrioventricular Nodal Reentrant Tachycardia (AVNRT)

This is a reentrant tachycardia that involves the AV node. The retrograde conduction typically occurs along the fast pathways. As a result, the atria are reactivated during or shortly after ventricular activation. During typical AVNRT, the P wave falls on the ST segment or within the terminal part of the QRS complex. (In most cases, the interval between ventricular and atrial activation—the V-A interval—is thus <70 ms) (Figs. 6.36 and 6.37).

Atrioventricular Reentrant Tachycardia (AVRT)

AVRT involves a circuit consisting of a slow anterograde conduit (composed of the atrium, the ventricle, and the AV node) and an accessory pathway that serves as the fast retrograde

Fig. 6.39 SVT with an approximate rate of 185 bpm, discernible P waves in V1 (*arrows*), and a VA of approximately 80 ms. The re-entry mechanism involves retrograde conduction along a concealed accessory pathway (absence of delta waves during sinus rhythm). The ST segment is also depressed (approximately 3 mm) in the precordial leads

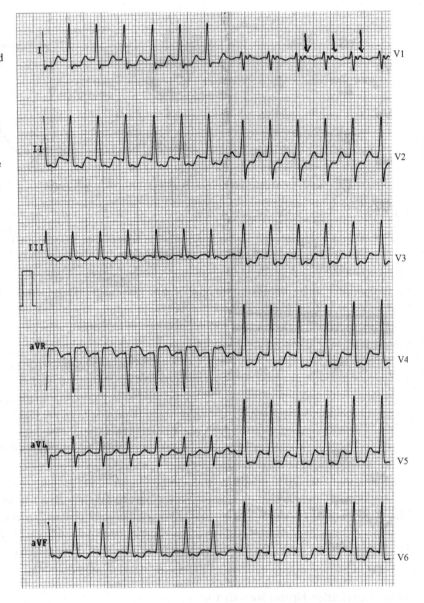

conduit. AVRT is also referred to as *orthodromic reciprocating tachycardia*. In approximately 15 % of cases, the abnormal pathway allows only retrograde conduction, and the classic delta wave (see Chap. 7) cannot be recorded in sinus rhythm. During tachycardia, an obvious atrial wave is recorded, especially by V1, with a V-A interval of >70 ms (Fig. 6.39). Additional characteristics of tachycardias related to accessory pathways can be found in Chap. 7.

Distinguishing between AVNRT and AVRT is not always easy. If P waves are missing (even in part), the most likely diagnosis is AVNRT. The P wave may be partly hidden within the QRS complex, which is thereby distorted. The result is a pseudo r′ wave in V1 (Fig. 6.35) and/or a pseudo-S wave in the inferior leads. These findings are highly indicative of AVNRT (reported accuracy 100 %). A discernible P wave in the ST segment with an R-P interval ≥70 ms is highly indicative of AVRT. Some authors (Riva et al.) maintain that ST depression of >2 mm in the precordial leads associated with T-wave inversion (reflecting retrograde activation of the atrium) is another distinguishing feature that supports a diagnosis of AVRT (Fig. 6.39).

Long-RP Tachycardias

A peculiar characteristic of the RP > PR tachycardias is the presence of negative P waves in the inferior leads. The differential diagnosis includes atypical AVNRT, permanent junctional reciprocating tachycardia (Coumel type PJRT) (a form of AVRT related to a slow, retrograde conduction through an accessory pathway, which is often located in the posteroseptal region) (Fig. 6.40), and atrial tachycardia. Distinguishing between these disorders has important implications for the initial management of the arrhythmia. The first two forms are both based on the mechanism of reentry and can be differentiated only with intracardiac electrophysiology studies, and both can be resolved with catheter ablation. In contrast, atrial tachycardia with a 1:1 conduction rate is usually caused by abnormal automaticity, and it can sometimes be managed with drug therapy alone. Interruption of the arrhythmia following vagal maneuvers or adenosine administration points to one of the first two forms. If these measures have no effect on the atrial cycle and the tachycardia persists with an increased AV ratio, reentry can be excluded and the tachycardia definitively classified as atrial (Fig. 6.41). Interruption of PJRT tends to be followed by rapid recurrence. This distinguishes it from atypical AVNRT, which is otherwise similar to PJRT in terms of the ECG presentation.

In the rare event that atrial activity with a 1:1 AV conduction rate is associated with a wide QRS complex, the diagnostic algorithm illustrated in Fig. 6.50 should still be used. Indeed, these findings may represent VT with retrograde 1:1 ventricular-atrial conduction, especially if the patient is taking antiarrhythmic drugs capable of modifying the heart rate and allowing ventriculoatrial conduction that would otherwise be impossible. The correct diagnosis obviously has important implications for the acute-phase management of the arrhythmia (Fig. 6.42).

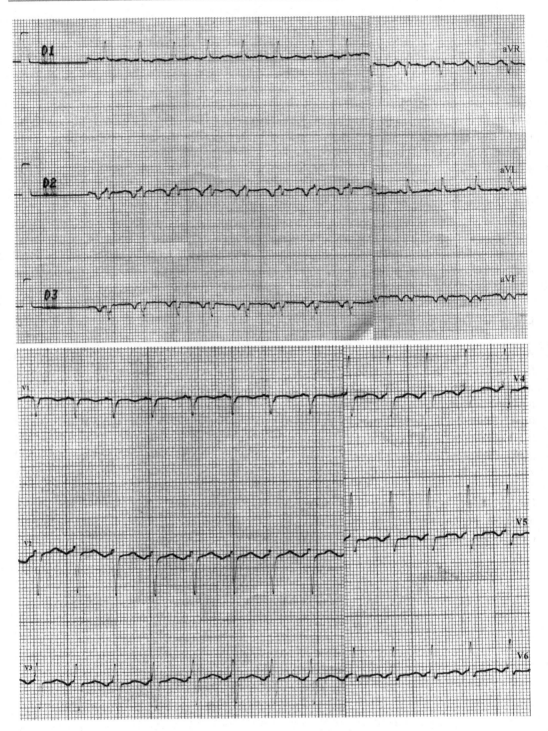

Fig. 6.40 PJRT with an approximate rate of 140 bpm. The P waves are negative in the inferior leads and the left precordial leads and positive in V1. The PR interval is 120 ms. Vagal maneuver interrupts the arrhythmia and restores sinus rhythm

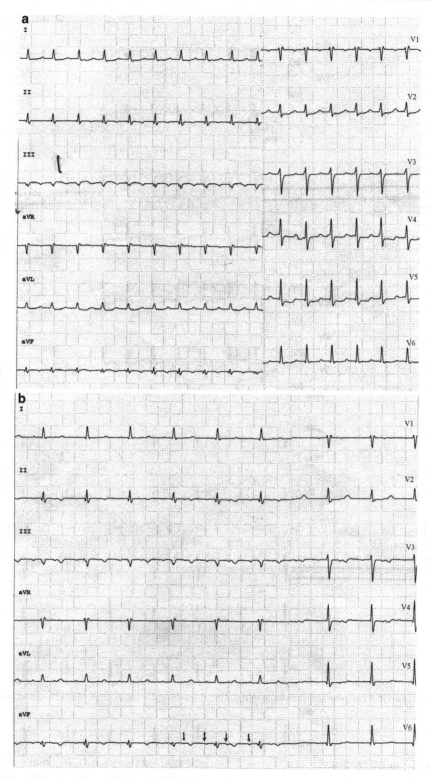

Fig. 6.41 (a) Tachycardia with RP > PR' pattern and incomplete RBBB conduction in a patient with a recent inferior myocardial infarction. In (b) vagal maneuver changes the AV ratio to 2:1 without interrupting the arrhythmia. The blocked P wave is in the ST segment, where its presence is reflected by the distortion of the repolarization wave (*vertical arrows* in lowermost tracing)

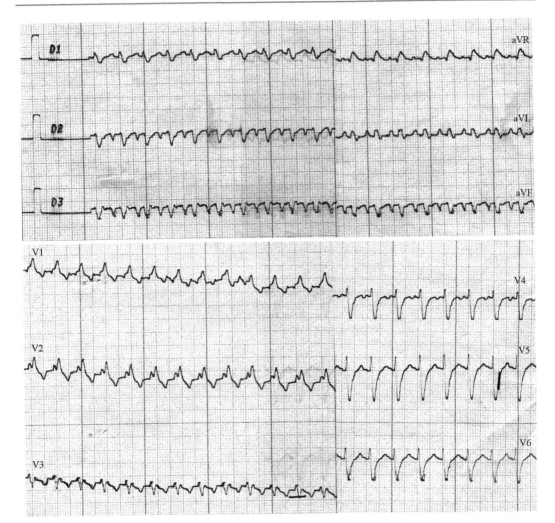

Fig. 6.42 Broad QRS complex RP > PR′ tachycardia with RBBB and LAFB. P waves are negative in the inferior leads but positive in V4, V5, and V6. The QRS complexes in the precordial leads exhibit a RBBB pattern with a QR complex in V1 and an R/S < 1 in V5-V6. The arrhythmia meets the Brugada criteria for a diagnosis of VT with specificity of >90 %. The Vi/Vt ratio (Vereckei criteria) is <1

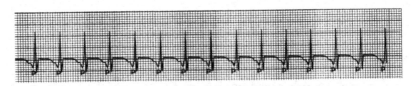

Fig. 6.43 Narrow QRS complex tachycardia with negative P waves and a PR interval of <120 ms, indicative of its junctional origin

Junctional Tachycardia

Junctional tachycardia is a nonparoxysmal form of long-RP tachycardia (Fig. 6.43) caused by increased automaticity. Its main electrocardiographic features are a PR interval of <120 ms and P-wave negativity in the inferior leads.

Differential Diagnosis of the Narrow-QRS-Complex Tachycardias

Distinguishing narrow-complex tachycardias from one another (Fig. 6.44) begins with the identification of the relation between atrial and ventricular activity (i.e., between the P wave and the QRS complex). P-wave morphology reflects the sequence of atrial activation. A P wave that is morphologically identical to that seen in sinus rhythm probably means that the tachycardia is originating somewhere near the SA node, regardless of the mechanism.

In the presence of morphological and temporal differences, there are two possibilities. In the first, the atrial activity precedes the QRS complex in a manner consistent with a normal atrioventricular delay. The RP interval in this case will be longer than the PR interval, the pattern typical of a long-RP tachycardia. The second possibility is that the P wave falls on or shortly after the QRS complex (i.e., on the ST-T segment), which suggests that the tachycardia is of the short-RP type.

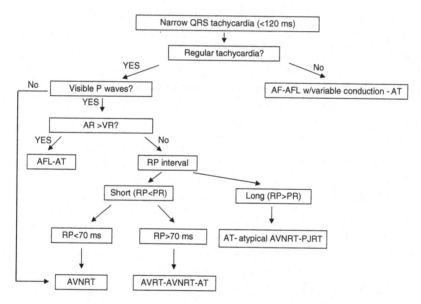

Fig. 6.44 Flow-chart for differential diagnosis of narrow-complex tachycardias. *AR* atrial rate, *VR* ventricular rate, *AF* atrial fibrillation, *AFL* atrial flutter, *AT* atrial tachycardia, *PJRT* permanent junctional reciprocating tachycardia, *AVNRT* atrioventricular nodal reentrant tachycardia, *AVRT* atrioventricular reentrant tachycardia

The Ventricular Arrhythmias

The ventricular arrhythmias include a wide variety of clinical-electrocardiographic entities, the simplest of which are the ventricular extrasystoles analyzed at the beginning of this chapter.

Monomorphic Ventricular Tachycardia

Ventricular tachycardia is defined as a tachyarrhythmia (rate >100 bpm) that tends to be regular and consists of at least 3 consecutive QRS complexes originating in one of the ventricles and a duration indicative of aberrant conduction (≥120 ms). Nonsustained VT lasts less than 30 seconds (Fig. 6.45). Sustained forms are those that last more than 30 seconds or that, regardless of their duration, produce hemodynamic instability and therefore require immediate termination.

The term *slow VT* is often used to refer to accelerated idioventricular rhythms (AIVRs), which are characterized by heart rates of 60–120 bpm. They are typically seen after acute myocardial infarction, when reperfusion has occurred (Fig. 6.46). When the infarction occurs

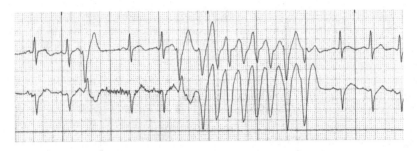

Fig. 6.45 Holter recording showing a short burst of nonsustained VT (approx. rate 200 bpm)

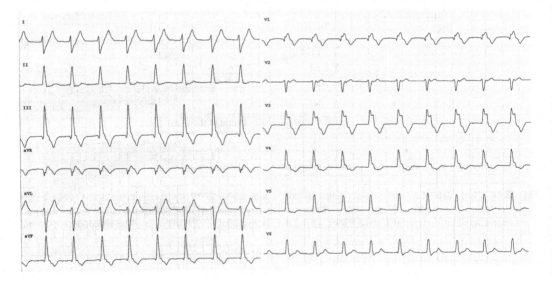

Fig. 6.46 Accelerated idioventricular rhythm during AMI. The QRS morphology is aberrant, the rate approximately 70 bpm, and atrioventricular dissociation is present. Typical reperfusion arrhythmia

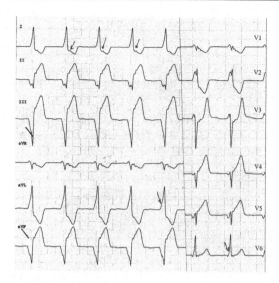

Fig. 6.47 ECG indicative of inferolateral AMI (ST-segment elevation in the inferior leads and in V4, V5, and V6) and morphologically complex, aberrantly conducted (duration: 160 ms) QRS complexes, which are suggestive of fusion between the ventricular and pre-excitation complexes. In fact, delta waves are clearly seen in leads I, aVL, and V6, along with retrograde conduction of the P waves from the ventricles to the atria (*vertical arrows* in lead I)

in a patient with ventricular pre-excitation, the AIVRs display alterations that are highly singular (Fig. 6.47). The ventricular rate distinguishes AIVRs from idioventricular rhythms, bradyarrhythmias with rates of <60 bpm caused by AV blocks or reduced sinus rates with the emergence of wide-QRS-complex escape rhythms (Fig. 6.48).

In most cases the electrical activities of the atria and ventricles are completely independent from one another. This atrioventricular dissociation is a specific and sensitive diagnostic criterion for identifying arrhythmias originating in the ventricles. Sometimes, however, a P wave occurring outside the refractory period of the AV node manages to "capture" the ventricles, that is, to activate them before they are activated by the ectopic impulse (Fig. 6.49). In this case, the resulting QRS complex will be narrow. If the ventricular capture is incomplete, however, a fusion complex will be recorded with a

morphology midway between that of the normal and ectopic beats.

In fewer than 15 % of cases, there is no atrioventricular dissociation, and retrograde conduction occurs through the AV node or through an accessory pathway. The conduction ratio is generally 1:1 rate although Wenckebach patterns are seen in some cases.

It is important to recall, however, that wide-complex tachycardia is not always VT: other possibilities include:

1. a supraventricular rhythm conducted aberrantly to the ventricles (complete bundle-branch-block (BBB) configuration) (Fig. 6.36);
2. a variant form of atrioventricular reentrant tachycardia in which an accessory pathway is used for anterograde conduction of the impulse (see Chap. 7, Fig. 7.3);
3. a supraventricular arrhythmia with aberrant conduction in a patient receiving flecainide or propafenone (Fig. 6.31).

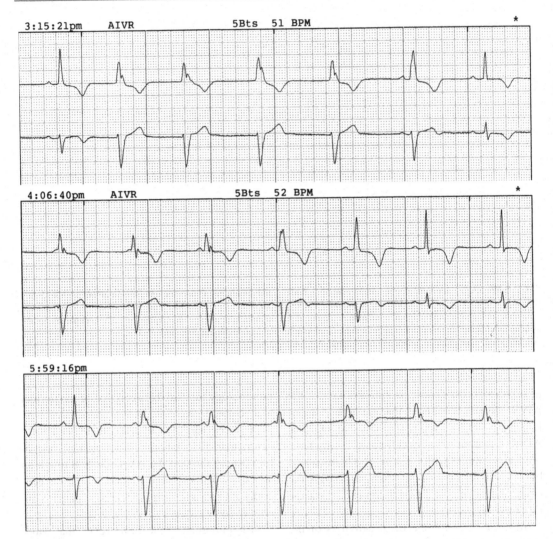

Fig. 6.48 Holter recording showing sinus bradycardia alternating with an idioventricular rhythm with a rate of 50 bpm, which is secondary to decreased sinus rate. Disappearance of the P waves can be observed along with progressive changes in the duration and morphology of the QRS complexes (fusion complexes)

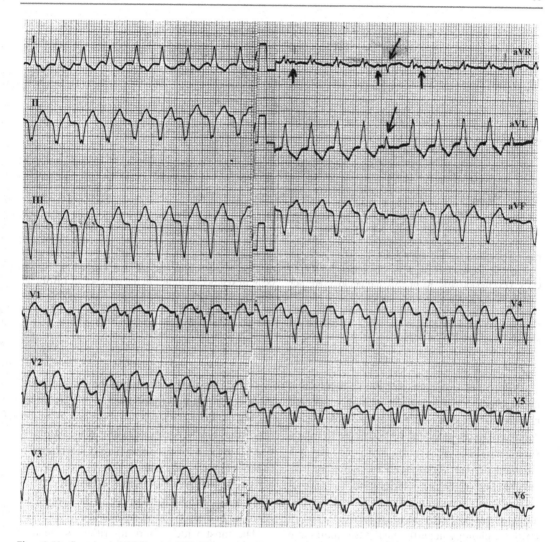

Fig. 6.49 Sustained LBBB-type VT. The precordial leads in the lower panel show QS-type ventricular complexes. In the unipolar limb leads (*upper panel* on the *right*), the 5th QRS complex (*downward-pointing arrows*) has a normal duration, and is preceded by a ventricle-capturing P wave. The *upward-pointing arrows* highlight the rate and activity of the P waves, which are completely dissociated from the ventricular complexes—all findings supporting a diagnosis of VT

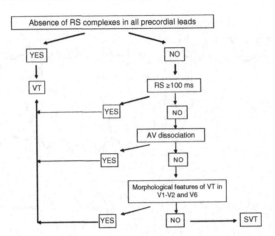

Fig. 6.50 Brugada algorithm for differential diagnosis of wide-QRS-complex tachycardias. Complexes with QR, QRS, QS, monophasic R, or rSR morphology are not considered RS complexes. In the presence of a RBBB-type QRS complex, one should consider the QRS morphology in V1 and the R/S ratio in V6: a triphasic complex in V1 and an R/S ratio of >1 in V6 is indicative of aberrancy, whereas other morphologies in V1, an R-wave duration of >30 ms in V1, and an R/S ratio of <1 in V6 point to ventricular forms. In the presence of LBBB, an RS interval of >60 ms, a Q wave in V6, and S-wave notching in V1 and V2 are indicative of VT. *AV* atrioventricular, *SVT* supraventricular tachycardia

Differential diagnosis has therapeutic implications for acute-phase management and prevention of recurrences. For example, using verapamil or propafenone or flecainide to treat a supraventricular tachycardia that is actually VT can have dramatic consequences, including irreversible hemodynamic deterioration.

To better understand the ECG criteria that allow correct differential diagnosis (analysis of QRS morphology in particular), it is important to recall that during aberrantly conducted SVT, activation of the septum occurs rapidly because it proceeds along the normal conduction pathways. The delay in ventricular activation involves the middle and terminal parts of the QRS. In contrast, the activation front in VT spreads more slowly at the beginning of the QRS complex until it reaches the His-Purkinje system. Thereafter, activation of the remaining portions of the ventricles occurs more rapidly.

Numerous diagnostic algorithms have been proposed based on criteria such as the electrical axes in the limb leads or QRS morphology in the precordial leads. Atrioventricular dissociation—that is, the electrocardiographically documented independence of atrial and ventricular activities—is the only one whose validity is undisputed, although it can be demonstrated in no more than 30 % of all cases.

The most widely used algorithm is the one proposed by Brugada et al. in 1991 and illustrated in Fig. 6.50. The sensitivity and specificity of this algorithm reported by the authors were 99 % and 96 %, respectively. The criteria related to the morphology of the QRS complexes in the precordial leads include: absence of RS complexes; or if such complexes are present, an RS interval of ≥100 ms; or in the presence of complete RBBB morphology, monophasic R or QR or RS complexes in V1.

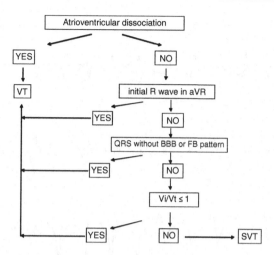

Fig. 6.51 Diagnostic algorithm proposed by Vereckei et al. *BBB* bundle-branch block, *FB* fascicular block

Later, however, the diagnostic capacity of the Brugada algorithm was challenged by some authors, in particular Vereckei et al. (Fig. 6.51). In 2007, they presented an algorithm that was similar to that of Brugada but specifically analyzed the aVR lead and the different components of the QRS complex. Lead aVR lies in the frontal plane at −210°, so if the electrical axis of the heart is within normal limits, it will record a negative QRS; a QRS complex consisting of an initial R wave alone in aVR indicates axis abnormality, like that which occurs in VT. For this reason, lead aVR can be considered the lead of reference for differential diagnosis of wide-complex tachycardias. Another criterion used for this purpose is related to the characteristics of VT-related ventricular activation described above. It consists in the assessment of the v_i:v_t ratio, where v_i is the conduction velocity measured in the first 40 milliseconds of a biphasic or multiphasic QRS complex and v_t is the velocity observed in the last 40 of the same complex. A v_i:v_t ratio of less than 1 is indicative of VT; a higher ratio points to SVT.

In 2010 Pava et al. proposed a new diagnostic criterion based on the analysis of the QRS complex in lead II: an interval of 50 ms or more between the onset of the QRS complex and the first peak of the R wave is highly indicative of VT (sensitivity 83 %). A recent comparison of this criterion and those of Vereckei (Vereckei 2014) showed the latter to be superior in terms of sensitivity and negative predictive power, whereas the former displayed greater specificity and a higher positive predictive power. The authors noted that in real-life clinical settings the diagnostic capacities of both criteria were inferior to those documented in the original studies. The point is that correct diagnosis of VT has to be based on integrated assessment of multiple criteria, and that the new algorithms that are really no more accurate than the classic criteria developed by Brugada.

The ECG examples proposed in the figures discussed below all come from cases of tachycardia in which the diagnosis was confirmed with electrophysiological studies.

Figure 6.49 shows tachycardia with a left bundle-branch block pattern and left axis deviation. This diagnosis can be made with both the Brugada and Vereckei algorithms since there are no RS complexes in any of

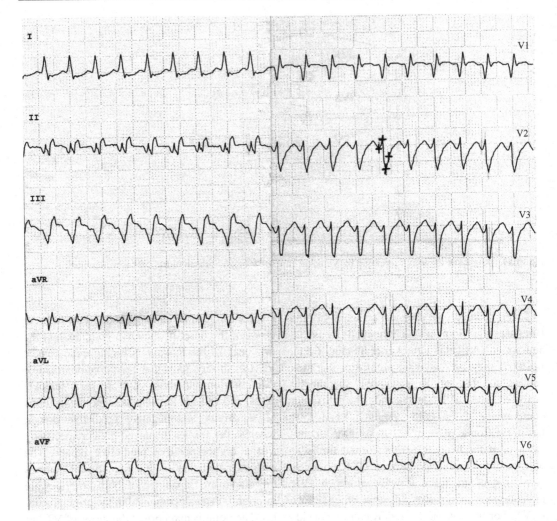

Fig. 6.52 VT with RBBB pattern and left axis deviation. The presence of the QR complex in V1 is one of the Brugada criteria for diagnosis of VT, but it is the one with the lowest specificity. In addition, the R/S ratio of <1 in not seen in V6, where there is an rsR′ complex. And finally, the RS complexes in the precordial leads have a duration of <100 ms. According to Vereckei, highly specific indicators of VT are the presence of an initial r wave in aVR and a Vi/Vt ratio of <1 in V2,V3, V4, or V5, where multiphasic complexes are more obvious and the initial and terminal components of the QRS complex are easier to identify

the precordial leads, and there is clear evidence of atrioventricular dissociation and ventricular capture. The case shown in Fig. 6.52 is less clear-cut: here the Brugada criteria are less stringently satisfied, whereas with the Vereckei criteria, the diagnosis of VT is straightforward. Atrioventricular dissociation is also evident in the tracings shown in Fig. 6.53, which meet all the criteria for VT using both approaches.

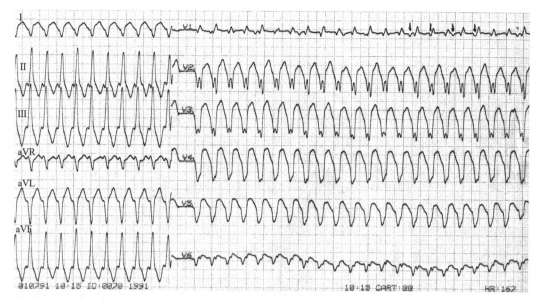

Fig. 6.53 RBBB-type VT with vertical axis. The *arrows* in V1 indicate the frequency of the P waves

Figure 6.54 shows a case of VT with a left bundle-branch block (LBBB) pattern: there are no RS complexes in the precordial leads, but V1 contains a triphasic QRS-like complex, and a large initial R wave is seen in aVR. Figure 6.55 also shows VT with a left BBB pattern and AV dissociation. RS complexes are present in the precordial leads with a duration of >100 ms.

In Fig. 6.56 the QRS morphology is indicative of a right bundle-branch block (RBBB) and a left anterior fascicular block (LAFB) (see Chap. 8), with a monophasic R wave in leads V1 and aVR and an R/S ratio of <1 in V6.

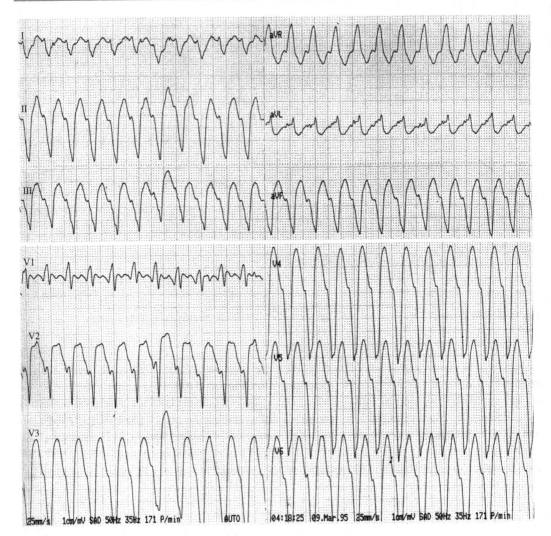

Fig. 6.54 LBBB-type VT. QRS in V1 but no RS complexes in the precordial leads. Large R wave in aVR. There may also be AV dissociation

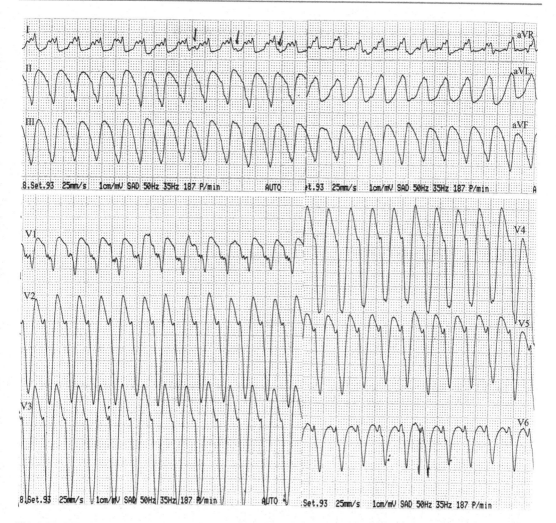

Fig. 6.55 VT with LBBB pattern. The diagnosis can be made with both algorithms. There is obvious AV dissociation (*arrows* in lead I), and the RS complexes in the precordial leads have a duration of >100 ms

The AV ratios in certain VTs are particularly interesting. In Fig. 6.57, for example, the pattern is that of a RBBB and LAFB. There appears to be atrioventricular dissociation. In all probability, however, there is actually some degree of retrograde ventriculoatrial conduction (3:1), as shown by the fact that the P-wave rate observed when sinus rhythm is restored is different from the P-wave rate during the VT.

Figure 6.58 shows VT with 1:1 retrograde conduction that was confirmed by the esophageal recording shown in Fig. 6.58b: the morphology of the QRS complex meets the criteria for VT in both algorithms.

VT occurs in many patients with chronic ischemic heart disease following a myocardial infarction. It is related to a reentry circuit at the boundary between scarred and viable zones of the myocardium. There are, however, less common forms that are associated with nonischemic heart disease (idiopathic dilated cardiomyopathy, valvular heart disease, the

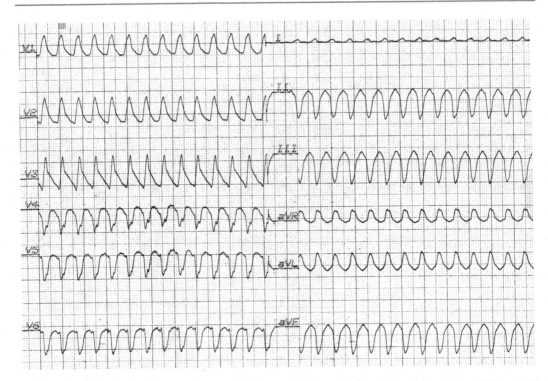

Fig. 6.56 VT with RBBB pattern and LAFB. The rapid rate makes it impossible to assess the possibility of AV dissociation. The R waves are monophasic in V1 and aVR, and the R/S ratio in V6 is <1

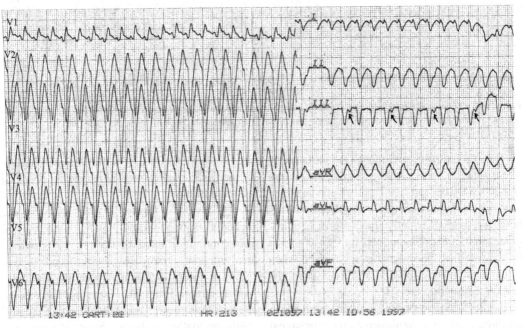

Fig. 6.57 VT with RBBB pattern and LAFB. In leads III and aVF, there are (*arrows*) negative P waves (caudocranial activation indicative of retrograde conduction), with a V-A ratio of 3:1. The QRS characteristics exclude the diagnosis of aberrant nodal tachycardia with a retrograde 3:1 block

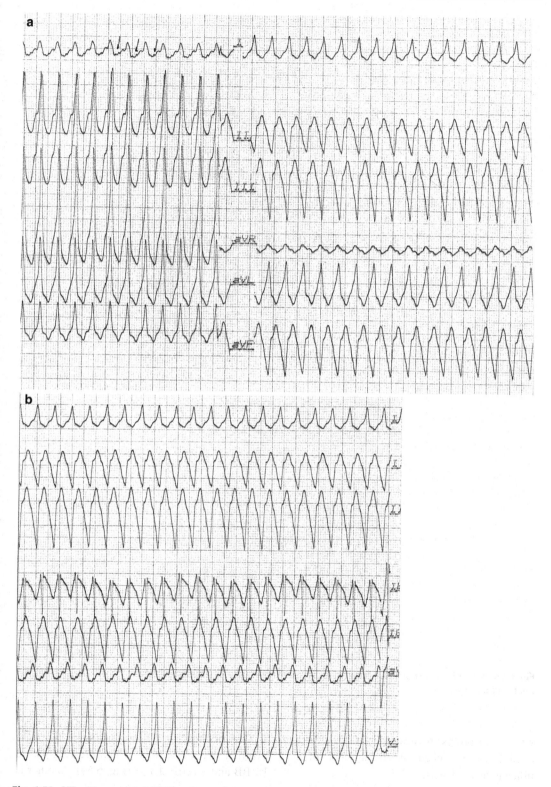

Fig. 6.58 VT with complete LBBB pattern and retrograde V-A conduction of 1:1 (**a**, **b**)

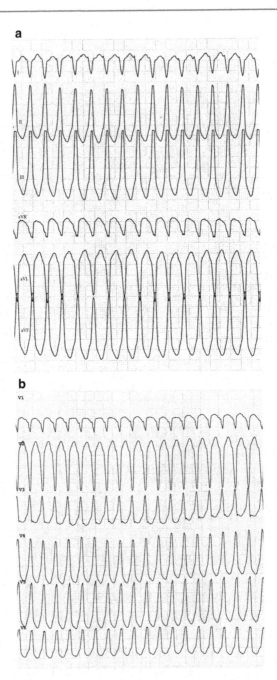

Fig. 6.59 VT with a LBBB pattern (origin in the RV) and a vertical axis (craniocaudal activation originating from the right ventricular outflow tract) (**a, b**)

genetic disorders reviewed in Chap. 8) and even some that occur in the absence of significant heart disease.

One of these is VT originating in the right ventricular outflow tract, which presents with a LBBB and a vertical axis (Fig. 6.59). Another is

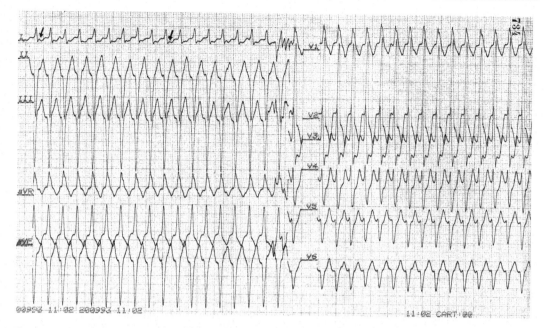

Fig. 6.60 An example of fascicular VT with a RBBB +LAFB pattern. The ventricular origin of the arrhythmia is suggested by several features: the presence of an R wave in aVR, the monophasic R wave configuration in V1, and the R/S ratio of <1 in V6. Careful observation of the ECG also reveals evidence of possible atrioventricular dissociation (*arrows*). Note that the duration of the QRS complex is only 120 ms

the form known as fascicular VT, which originates in one of the fascicles formed by the division of the left bundle branch or, less commonly, in the septal fascicles. The most frequent morphological pattern is RBBB+LAFB since the VT originates in the posterosuperior fascicle; the RBBB+LPFB (left posterior fascicular block) pattern is much less common. The distinctive feature of fascicular VT is its sensitivity to verapamil, which suggests that calcium-dependent fibers are involved in its development. The tachycardia is probably caused in part by a reentry circuit that causes base-to-apex activation of the interventricular septum (Fig. 6.60).

Other wide-complex tachycardias with more complex differential diagnoses are also shown. The one shown in Fig. 6.61, for example, is characterized by a complete left BBB and might be misdiagnosed as a supraventricular tachycardia with aberrancy. The correct diagnosis is based on examination of the V2 tracing, which meets the Brugada and Vereckei criteria for a ventricular arrhythmia.

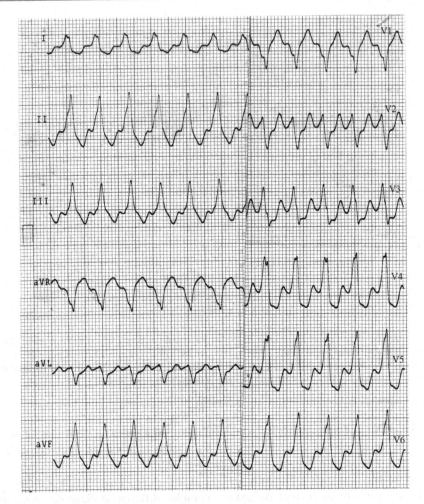

Fig. 6.61 VT with a complete LBBB pattern and a semivertical electrical axis. The morphology of the QRS in the precordial leads is initially suggestive of SVT with aberrancy, but analysis of the tracing from V2 shows an RS interval of 120 ms and a v_i/v_t ratio of 0.4, which is more indicative of an arrhythmia originating in the ventricles

Figure 6.62 shows VT with a RBBB and LAFB pattern. Clues to the diagnosis are the monophasic complex in the precordial leads and the initial r wave in aVR.

Finally, it is important to recall the possibility illustrated in Fig. 6.31: that a tachycardia with a QRS morphology that is unequivocally typical of VT may actually be secondary to atrial flutter in a patient receiving class IC antiarrhythmic drugs.

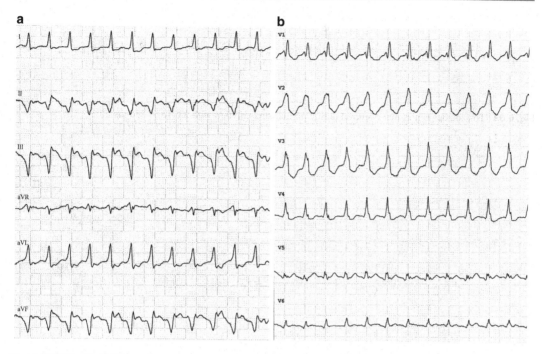

Fig. 6.62 VT with RBBB pattern and LAFB (**a, b**). The QRS complexes are essentially monophasic in the precordial leads with an r wave in aVR. Atrioventricular dissociation is probably also present

Polymorphic Ventricular Tachycardia

This morphologically distinctive form of VT is characterized by continuous, phasic variation of the polarity of the QRS complex, which appears to "twist" around the isoelectric line: hence the term *torsade de pointes* (TdP) (Fig. 6.63). It is a potentially life-threatening arrhythmia: in some cases, it occurs in self-limiting runs lasting a few seconds, which are associated with syncopal or presyncopal symptoms, but in others—by no means rare—it leads to a sudden, fatal cardiac arrest. In most cases, the arrhythmia has specific, correctable causes associated with significant prolongation of the QT interval. The latter is a reflection of markedly inhomogeneous ventricular repolarization, which is the primary electrical event in the genesis of this arrhythmia. The main causes include:

1. the congenital long-QT syndrome, which is discussed in detail in Chap. 8;
2. electrolyte disturbances, in particular hypokalemia and hypomagnesemia;
3. antiarrhythmic drug therapy, especially with drugs of class IA (quinidine, procainamide, disopyramide) or IC (amiodarone, sotalol);
4. noncardiovascular drug therapy (see Chap. 9, Table 9.1).

Torsade de pointes VT is often associated with bradyarrhythmias (any origin) characterized by significant QT prolongation and R-on-T premature ventricular complexes, which trigger the

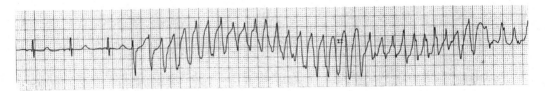

Fig. 6.63 Torsade de pointes that occurred during normal sinus rhythm with a QTc of 530 ms

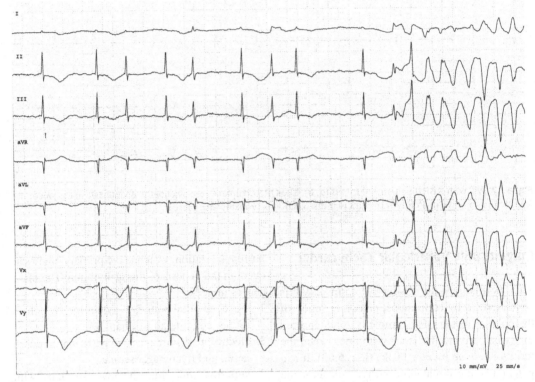

Fig. 6.64 Torsade de pointes VT in a patient with AF and long QT syndrome. The arrhythmia lasted approximately 20 seconds and was preceded by a long RR cycle

lasting 1240 ms, much longer than that of the previous complex. The phenomenon recurs in all complexes the end long cycles

arrhythmia, typically after a long RR cycle (Figs. 6.64 and 6.65). The bradycardia causes QT interval prolongation and dispersion of ventricular refractoriness, thereby facilitating onset of the arrhythmia. This can occur during sinus or junctional bradycardia, bradycardia caused by complete AV block. The mechanism is thought to be related to early afterdepolarizations (see Chap. 4), which are in fact bradycardia-dependent and secondary to significant prolongation of the action potential.

A less common variant is polymorphic VT with a normal QT interval and no evidence of structural heart disease. The main

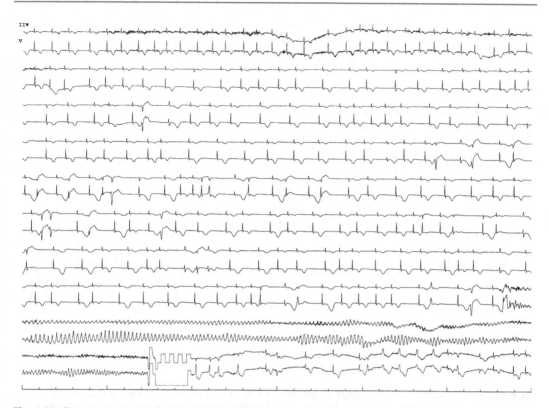

Fig. 6.65 Torsade de pointes with behavior similar to that seen in Fig. 6.64

electrocardiographic characteristics is a short cycle between the last normal QRS complex and that of the first ectopic ventricular beat (Fig. 6.66); unlike TdP, this variant can rarely be attributed to a specific, reversible cause. The most commonly reported mechanism is related to delayed, calcium-dependent afterdepo-larizations, but the rate increase right before the appearance of the arrhythmia is thought to be a contributing factor (increased adrenergic tone). The tachyarrhythmic episodes can often be successfully controlled with calcium-channel blockers, as in the case illustrated in Fig. 6.66.

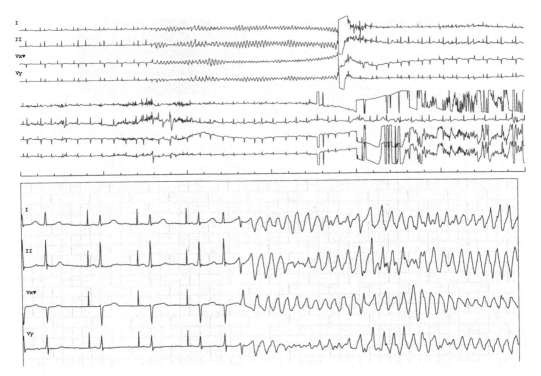

Fig. 6.66 Polymorphic VT with a normal QT in a patient with a dual-chamber defibrillator. The ECG shows one of the recurrent episodes experienced by the patient, all triggered in the same way: the baseline pacing rhythm (AAI mode, rate: 60 bpm, normal QTc of 400 ms) is interrupted by an atrial extrasystole, which triggers the VT. Possible association between late afterdepolarizations and increased adrenergic tone

Ventricular Fibrillation

Ventricular fibrillation is the most dangerous of all the arrhythmias, in that it is invariably fatal, but it is also one of the easiest to recognize. Its chaotic oscillations vary widely in frequency and amplitude, and the normal components of the tracing, including the isoelectric line, are unrecognizable (Fig. 6.67). Direct-current (DC) shock is the only way to terminate it (Fig. 6.68).

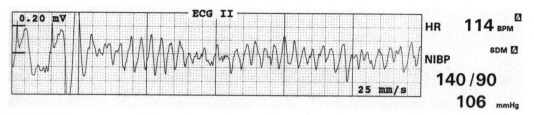

Fig. 6.67 Ventricular fibrillation triggered by a premature VEB during acute myocardial infarction (ST-segment elevation)

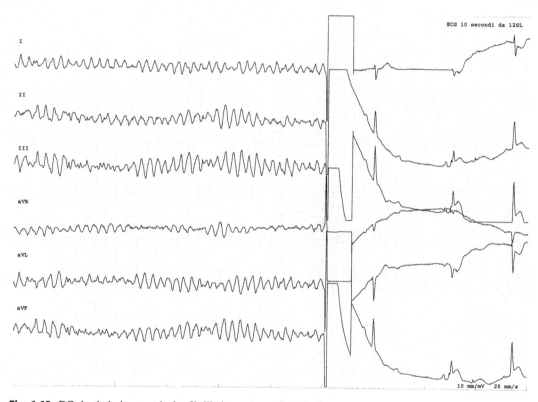

Fig. 6.68 DC shock during ventricular fibrillation restores sinus rhythm

The Electrocardiogram in Wolff-ParkinsonWhite Syndrome

7

Introduction

In its most common form, the Wolff-Parkinson-White (WPW) syndrome is caused by the presence of an embryonic remnant consisting of an accessory atrioventricular pathway. When the pathway bypasses the AV node and connects the atria directly to the ventricles, it is referred to as the bundle of Kent. Less frequently, the anomalous connection is between the AV node or bundle of His and the ventricles, and it is referred to as the bundle of Mahaim. The bundle of Kent is by far the more common variant. In this case, the excitation wavefront travels simultaneously through the usual pathway (the AV node, which normally slows conduction) and much more rapidly through the accessory pathway, thereby activating the ventricles earlier than usual. As a result, the P-R interval is shortened, and the initial part of the ventricular complex is slurred or notched. This distortion is referred to as a *delta wave*, and it is pathognomonic for the WPW syndrome. The QRS complex in this case is actually a fusion of the complexes resulting from the two pathways of ventricular activation (Figs. 7.1 and 7.2).

The accessory pathway may be located in the free wall of the left or right ventricle or in the interventricular septum. In some cases, there may be more than one. In around 15 % of cases, it conducts exclusively in a retrograde direction and is referred to as a *concealed* accessory pathway. Preexcitation has been historically classified as type A or type B (although this distinction of limited value). Accessory pathways located in the left side of the heart give rise to type A preexcitation, with premature activation of the left ventricle. The QRS complexes in this case are generally positive in the right precordial leads and exhibit a right bundle-branch-block (RBBB) pattern. Right-heart pathways produce type B preexcitation, with premature activation of the right ventricle and QRS complexes with a left bundle-branch-block (LBBB) morphology. When type-B pathways are located posteriorly, they often give rise to Q waves or QS complexes in leads II, III, and aVF, findings that can be misinterpreted as signs of an inferior myocardial infarction. The exact location of the accessory pathway cannot always be determined on the basis of surface electrocardiographic findings. Diagnostic algorithms have been developed for this purpose although their sensitivity and specificity varies (Fig. 7.3). In general, the delta-wave vector is directed away from the ventricular zone that is pre-excited by the accessory pathway (Table 7.1).

The WPW syndrome may be asymptomatic or associated with supraventricular tachyarrhythmias, such as paroxysmal supraventricular reciprocating tachycardia (80 %), atrial fibrillation (AF) (15 %), or atrial flutter (5 %) (see

M. Romanò, *Text Atlas of Practical Electrocardiography*, DOI 10.1007/978-88-470-5741-8_7, © Springer-Verlag Italia 2015

Fig. 7.1 *Right*: Diagram of the Kent bundle-type accessory conduction pathway and typical ECG showing a delta wave. *Left*: Diagram pf the normal excitation-conduction system and normal ECG

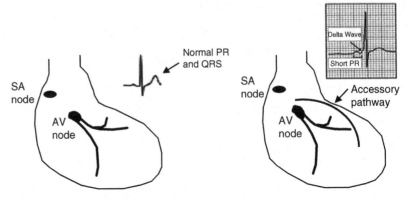

Fig. 7.2 ECG showing left ventricular preexcitation: sinus rhythm (rate 70 bpm), short PR interval (0.08 s), QRS duration 0.12 s. The delta wave is positive in the precordial leads and in aVF with an intermediate electrical axis in the frontal plane

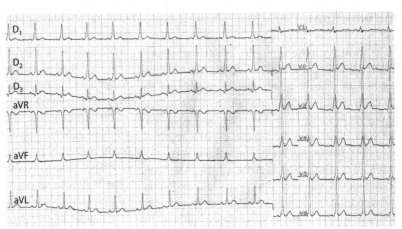

Fig. 7.3 Algorithm for localization of the accessory pathway

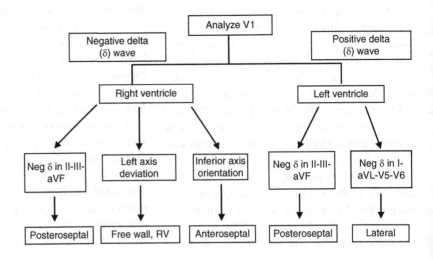

Table 7.1 General criteria for localizing the accessory pathway

Free wall of the left ventricle
positive delta wave in V1 (R/S>1): if the delta wave is positive in aVF, the pathway is probably located in the lateral or anterolateral wall; an isoelectric or negative delta wave points to the posterior or posterolateral wall
Left posteroseptal region
delta waves that are positive in most precordial leads and negative in the inferior leads
Right anteroseptal region
delta waves that are negative in V1-V2 and positive in aVF
Right posteroseptal region
delta waves that are negative in V1 and in the inferior leads
Free wall of the right ventricle
delta waves that are negative in V1-V2 and positive in leads I and V6

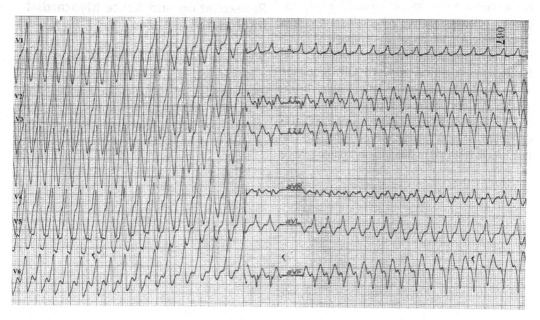

Fig. 7.4 Example of paroxysmal antidromic reentrant SVT (rate 180 bpm). The QRS complexes are broad, but their ventricular origin is excluded by the obvious delta wave in the precordial leads (left-hand tracing)

Chap. 6). Supraventricular tachycardia (SVT) triggered by atrial or ventricular extrasystoles is sustained by a re-entry circuit composed of the atrium, AV node, one of the ventricles, and the accessory pathway (Fig. 6.38). The tachycardia is described as *orthodromic* when the AV node serves as the anterograde conduit of the circuit and the accessory pathway provides retrograde conduction. The QRS complex is generally narrow in this case, unless there is a functional bundle branch block. Not uncommonly, this form of SVT is sustained by a concealed accessory pathway, that is, one that conducts exclusively from the ventricles toward the atria. For this reason, the delta waves are not visible on the ECG during sinus rhythm. A concealed accessory pathway should be suspected when the QRS complex during tachycardia is normal in morphology and followed by a P wave that falls within the ST segment or the initial portion of the T wave (Fig. 6.39). The interval between onset of the QRS and onset of this P wave generally exceeds 70 ms (i.e., longer than the V-A interval seen in SVT caused by nodal re-entry—see Chap. 6). If, instead, the accessory pathway is the anterograde conduit and retrograde conduction occurs through the AV node, the SVT is said to be *antidromic*, and the QRS morphology is characterized by a delta wave and aberrancy reflecting total preexcitation (Fig. 7.4). This form is less common.

Atrial Fibrillation and Ventricular Preexcitation

AF in the presence of an accessory pathway is associated with singular clinical and electrocardiographic features. The accessory pathway generally has a longer refractory period than the AV node, so during AF the impulse passes preferentially through the node itself, and the QRS complex resembles that seen during sinus rhythm. Less commonly, the accessory pathway has a shorter refractory period and higher conduction velocity than the AV node, and in this case, during AF, the impulse is propagated to the ventricles through the accessory pathway. The ECG shows a typical widened QRS complex with variable aberrancy. This latter feature distinguishes AF associated with pre-excitation from AF conducted with a BBB, which is also characterized by a broad QRS complex but one that is constant in duration and morphology (see Chap. 6, Fig. 6.19). Variable duration of the QRS complex reflects the fact that the electrical impulse is being propagated wholly or in part via the accessory pathway (Fig. 7.5). In these cases, the ventricular response can be as high as 300 bpm, and the arrhythmia may well degenerate into ventricular fibrillation causing sudden death.

Less commonly, preexcitation is associated with atrial flutter (Fig. 7.6).

Preexcitation and Acute Myocardial Infarction

When acute myocardial infarction occurs against a background of ventricular pre-excitation, the ECG findings are singular. The example shown in Fig. 7.7 includes ST segment elevation in the inferior and lateral leads and QRS aberrancy suggestive of an accessory conduction pathway.

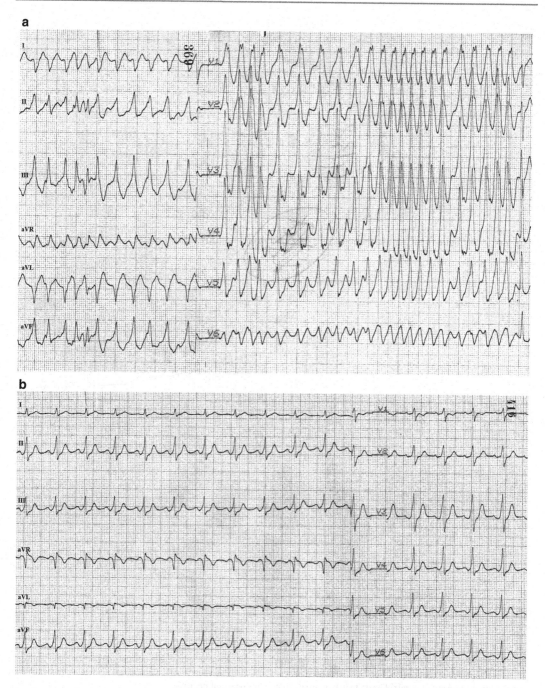

Fig. 7.5 (a) AF in the presence of ventricular preexcitation with AV conduction via an accessory pathway. P waves are absent, the ventricular response is very rapid (mean: 220 bpm, maximum: 290 bpm) and irregular, and the QRS complexes are wide with varying degrees of aberrancy. (This variability is the hallmark of ventricular pre-excitation.) (b) Same patient after restoration of sinus rhythm. ECG findings indicative of a left-sided accessory pathway, probably in the lateral wall

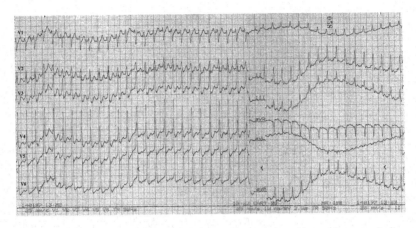

Fig. 7.6 Atrial flutter with 2:1 conduction and QRS morphology indicative of incomplete ventricular preexcitation

a

b

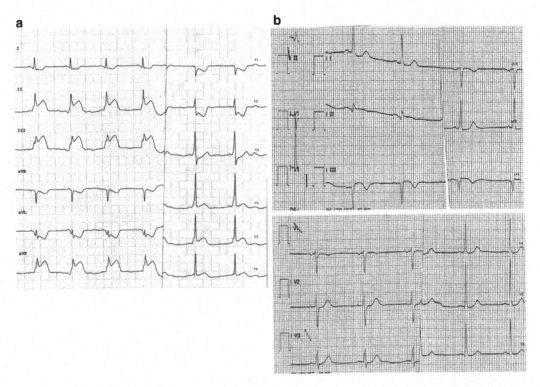

Fig. 7.7 (a) Acute inferolateral myocardial infarction with ventricular preexcitation caused by a left-sided accessory pathway (probably lateral). The delta waves are visible mainly in the left precordial leads. (b) The QRS complexes in the subacute phase are normal in morphology, but there is clear evidence of inferolateral Q waves indicative of myocardial necrosis

Bundle-Branch Blocks and Fascicular Blocks

8

Intraventricular Conduction Delays: General Principles

For a review of the anatomy of the His-Purkinje network, see Chap. 1.

Bundle-branch blocks (BBBs) and fascicular blocks (also referred to as hemiblocks) are disturbances involving the electrical activation of the ventricles. As the terms suggest, the conduction impairment usually occurs in the bundle branches or their fascicles, but blocks may also be located in the bundle of His or in the most peripheral branches of the conduction network. Bundle-branch blocks are manifested on the electrocardiogram (ECG) by widening of the QRS complex and may be complete (QRS duration of >120 ms) or incomplete (QRS duration between 110 and 120 ms). The abnormal ventricular depolarization causes secondary changes in the repolarization phase, including inversion of the T waves in leads where they are normally positive and sometimes ST-segment depression.

Bundle-branch blocks can be permanent or temporary, regressing, that is, when the conditions that generated them (e.g., acute ischemia, acute cor pulmonale) begin to improve.

They can also be described as stable or intermittent. The latter forms usually appear when the heart rate increases (rate-dependent bundle-branch blocks).

Right Bundle-Branch Block

In the presence of a right bundle-branch block (RBBB), the interventricular septum depolarizes normally, from left to right, and the left ventricle is also activated normally. In contrast, depolarization of the right ventricle is delayed since the right ventricle is the last to be activated. The widening of the QRS complex is largely due to the delayed activation of the right side of the septum and free wall of the right ventricle.

The typical ECG features of RBBB are recorded in lead V1. The normal activation of the septum is inscribed as a large R wave followed by an S wave, which reflects activation of the left ventricle, and a terminal R' wave representing delayed right ventricular depolarization proceeding anteriorly and to the right (Fig. 8.1). The depth of the S wave in lead V1 varies depending on whether the left ventricular activation vector is

M. Romanò, *Text Atlas of Practical Electrocardiography*, DOI 10.1007/978-88-470-5741-8_8, © Springer-Verlag Italia 2015

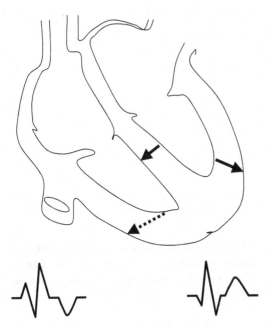

Fig. 8.1 Diagram showing the altered sequence of ventricular activation during complete RBBB. The *solid arrows* indicate preserved activation of the interventricular septum and the free wall of the left ventricle. The *dotted arrow* highlights the delayed activation of the right side of the interventricular septum and free wall of the right ventricle

oriented posteriorly or anteriorly. In the former case, the R and R′ waves will be separated by a prominent S wave; in the latter case, the S wave may be small, slurred, or completely absent (Figs. 8.2 and 8.3). The leads facing the left side of the septum (I, aVL, V5, and V6) will record an initial q wave followed by an R wave of normal duration and an S wave that is wide and relatively shallow. A late R wave will be present in lead aVR, reflecting delayed activation of the right ventricle.

In the presence of a RBBB, the mean axis of the QRS complex in the frontal plane is generally normal. In some cases, there is a right deviation of 15°–30°, but the axis is often indeterminate.

The altered ventricular depolarization process leads to changes in the repolarization phase as well. The direction of the T wave will be opposite to that of the terminal component of the QRS complex, that is, positive in lead I, where the ventricular complex ends with an S wave, and negative in V1, where the terminal wave is an R

or R′. If this relation is not maintained, the repolarization abnormality is probably primary rather than secondary.

Since the most diagnostically significant elements of the QRS complex are unaltered in RBBB, normality and abnormality can be defined by criteria related to voltage, R-wave progression, and Q waves: RBBB does not interfere with the diagnosis of left ventricular hypertrophy (LVH) or myocardial infarction (Figs. 8.2–8.4).

Left Bundle-Branch Block

In left bundle-branch block (LBBB), conduction is delayed at the level of the left bundle branch, proximal to its division into anterior and posterior fascicles. It reverses the direction of depolarization in the interventricular septum and delays activation of the free wall of the left ventricle. In some cases (the minority), the delay occurs in the bundle of His, but the fibers destined to form the two bundle branches are already separate at this level, so these cases are really no different from true LBBB.

Interruption of conduction at the level of the left bundle branch causes premature activation of the right side of the septum and the right ventricular myocardium. Right-to-left trans-septal activation occurs through the ventricular myocardium and is a slow process. It is probably the main cause of the prolonged ventricular activation. In fact, a complete block within the left bundle branch delays depolarization of the free wall of the left ventricle and decreases its velocity, but its most important effect is reversal of the direction in which the interventricular septum is depolarized.

This produces obvious changes in the electrocardiogram, which involve the direction of the initial deflection in the QRS complex. Leads that formerly recorded an initial r wave now record a q wave; those normally showing an initial q wave now exhibit an r wave (Fig. 8.5).

These two alterations cause typical changes in the precordial leads: the QRS morphology is completely altered in both V1 and in V6. The fundamental ECG features are the absence of the

Fig. 8.2 ECG recording from a patient with severe arterial hypertension and a complete RBBB. In lead V1 there is an rsR′ complex and in leads V6 and I a delayed prominent S wave. The electrical axis is semivertical. The T wave is positive in lead I and negative in V1. Small q waves are present in the leads exploring the left ventricle. The tracing meets the voltage criteria for left ventricular hypertrophy associated with left atrial enlargement

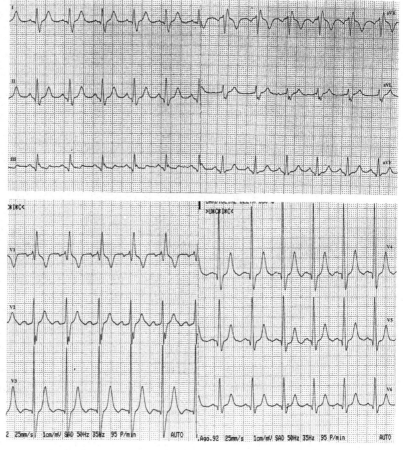

Fig. 8.3 RBBB associated with LAFB. An RR' complex is present in lead V1

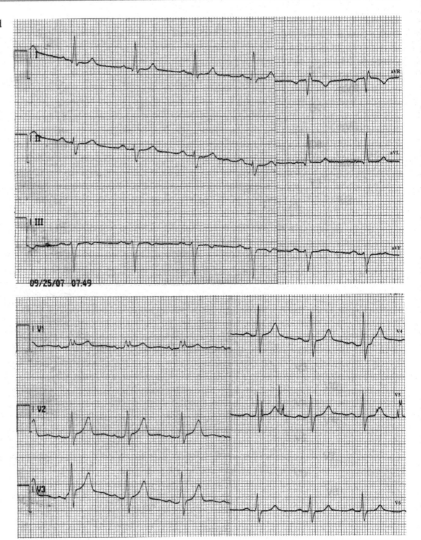

Fig. 8.4 ECG showing acute myocardial infarction of the anterior wall with complete RBBB and left axis deviation, which can be easily diagnosed on the basis of the QR complexes in V1, the RS complexes in leads I and aVL, and the Rs complexes in lead V6

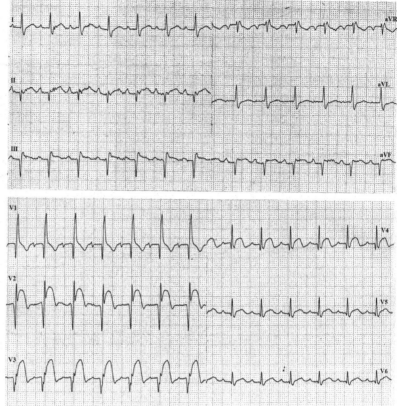

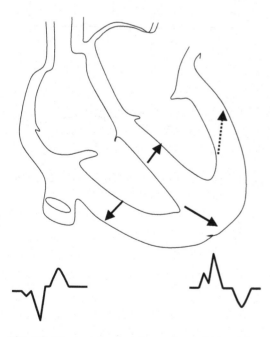

Fig. 8.5 Diagram showing abnormal ventricular activation during complete LBBB. Right ventricular activation is unchanged, but the direction of activation is reversed in the septum and free wall of the left ventricle

septal q wave in lead V6 and prolongation of the QRS complex.

The results are deep QS complexes in leads V1 and V2 and broad notched or slurred R waves in leads V5, V6, I and aVL (Fig. 8.6). The mean QRS axis in the frontal plane may be normal or deviated, usually to the left (from −30° to −90°), less commonly to the right (Fig. 8.7). The direction of the QRS vector is opposite to those of the ST segment and T wave. Positive QRS complexes in leads I, aVL, and V6 will therefore be associated with depressed ST segments and negative T waves, whereas in leads V1, V2 and V3, where predominantly negative QRS complexes are seen, ST-segment elevation or positive T waves will be found. The ST and T wave changes are secondary to the impaired conduction, and the magnitude of the alterations is proportional to the degree of QRS aberrancy (Fig. 8.8).

The ST-segment and T-wave changes associated with complete LBBB can mask signs of myocardial ischemia and acute myocardial

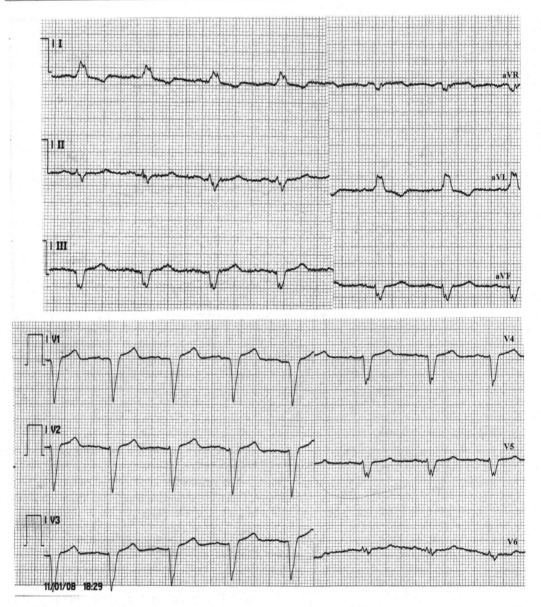

Fig. 8.6 Complete LBBB with left axis deviation. Note the broad and notched QRS complex (160 ms) in leads I, aVL, and V6

Fig. 8.7 Complete LBBB with right axis deviation (+150°) in a patient with dilated cardiomyopathy

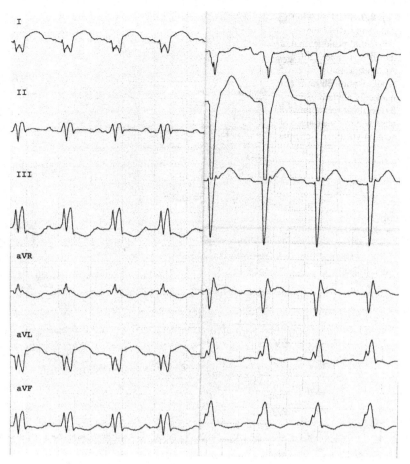

Fig. 8.8 ECG showing complete LBBB with substantial prolongation of the QRS complex (220 ms). As a result, the repolarization phase is also markedly altered: ST-segment elevation is observed in the absence of acute myocardial ischemia

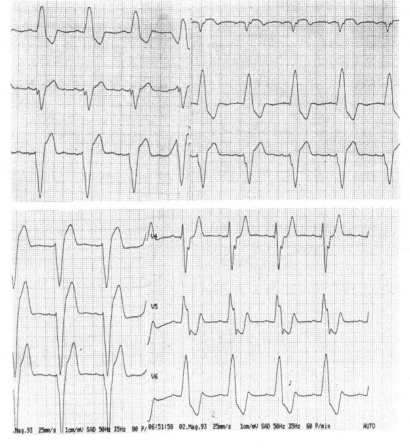

infarction, thereby rendering the diagnosis more difficult.

In the presence of a LBBB, right ventricular activation precedes left ventricular activation. When myocardial infarction occurs, activation of the necrotic area in the left ventricle is delayed, and it is obscured within the QRS complex. Therefore, the classic Q wave is absent and cannot be used to diagnose infarction. In the earliest phases of the infarction, the ST-segment concordance criteria proposed in 1996 by Sgarbossa et al. are independent predictors of acute myocardial ischemia in the presence of a LBBB:

– ST-segment elevation of ≥1 mm in a lead with a positive QRS complex (directional concordance between the major QRS-complex and ST-segment vectors);
– ST segment depression of ≥1 mm in lead V1, V2, or V3;
– ST segment depression of ≥1 mm in leads II, III, and aVF and ST segment elevation of ≥1 mm in lead V5;
– ST segment elevation of ≥5 mm in the presence of a negative QRS complex (extreme directional discordance between QRS and ST-segment vectors) (Fig. 8.9).

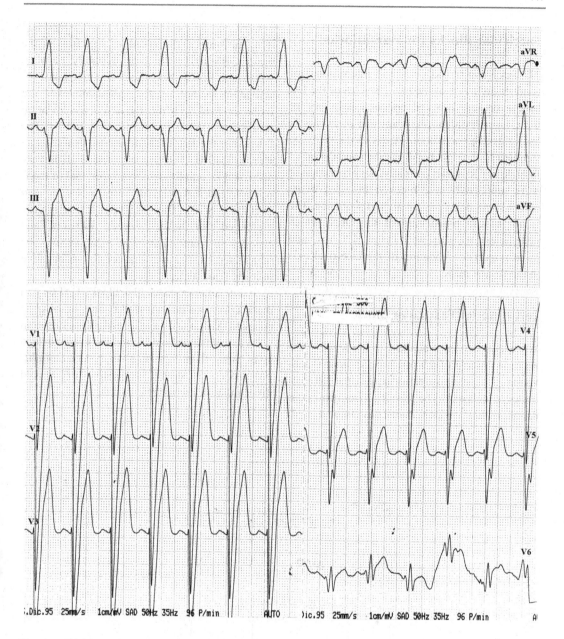

Fig. 8.9 ECG in a patient with complete LBBB (QRS duration 160 ms, rS complex in V1 and polyphasic complex in V6, left axis deviation) and signs of an acute anterior myocardial infarction. In leads V1, V2, V3, and V4, ST-segment elevation >10 mm is present, fulfilling the Sgarbossa criteria

Fascicular Blocks (or Hemiblocks)

The fascicular blocks consist in interruptions of conduction in one of the two fascicles of the left bundle branch. Blocked conduction in one of these fascicles alters the sequence of events in left ventricular activation. Areas of the ventricle supplied by the right bundle branch and the intact fascicle are activated normally, depolarization of parts supplied by the blocked fascicle occurs with a slight delay and an altered sequence. The result is mild broadening of the QRS, which nonetheless remains well below 120 ms, and more important, deviation of the electrical axis in the frontal plane.

Left Anterior Fascicular Block

When conduction is blocked at the level of the anterior fascicle of the left bundle branch, activation of the anterosuperior part of the left ventricle is delayed. The result is asynchronous depolarization, which translates into a shift upward and to the left in the intermediate and terminal forces and marked left deviation of the mean QRS axis (which is normally between −30° and −60°). Because the initial phase of activation is not altered, qR complexes are found in lead I, while the left axis deviation results in rS complexes in leads II and III. The S wave in the latter lead is deeper than the one seen in lead II. The S wave in lead III is very deep, and its amplitude may exceed that of the R wave in lead I. A delayed r′ wave is seen in lead aVR (Fig. 8.10). The QRS complex is slightly prolonged but never exceeds 120 ms, and changes in ventricular repolarization may be manifested by T waves that are flat or negative in leads I and aVL.

A left anterior fascicular block (LAFB) can mask a previous inferior wall infarct. In the presence of LAFB, the r wave in lead aVF is higher in voltage that that in lead III, and the r wave in lead II is taller than that in aVF: reversal of this progression is highly suggestive of an old myocardial infarction (Fig. 8.11).

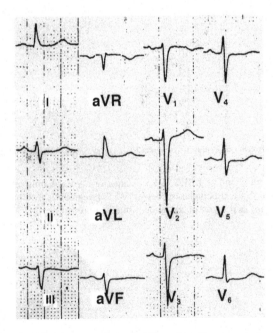

Fig. 8.10 Left axis deviation (−30°), late r wave in lead aVR, and small q wave in leads I and aVL

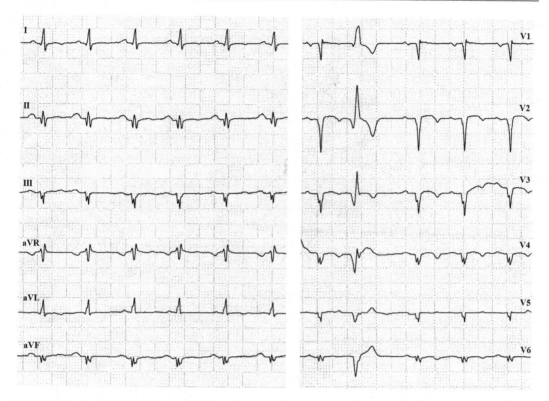

Fig. 8.11 Results of a simultaneous anterior and inferior myocardial infarction (U infarction). The limb leads (*left*) show LAFB and evidence of the inferior infarct (q wave in lead II and small r wave in lead III with higher voltage than that of the r wave in lead aVF)

Left Posterior Fascicular Block

Delayed conduction through the posterior fascicle of the left ventricle causes a downward shift in the intermediate and terminal forces of left ventricular activation. As a result, the mean QRS axis in the frontal plane becomes vertical and shifts to the right (past +90°), rS-type complexes are seen in lead I, qR-type complexes in leads II and III (the R in lead III is taller than that in lead II), r waves are small or absent in aVR, and s waves are small or absent in leads V5 and V6 (Fig. 8.12).

These criteria are valid only when right ventricular hypertrophy can be excluded since it

produces similar changes in the electrical axis. In addition, right deviation of the mean QRS complex (+110° and beyond) may be normal in adolescents and children.

Bifascicular Blocks

Conduction delays involving two fascicles (i.e., the right bundle branch and the left anterior or left posterior fascicle) are referred to as bifascicular. The changes that can be recorded on ECG are the sum of the alterations produced by the individual blocks.

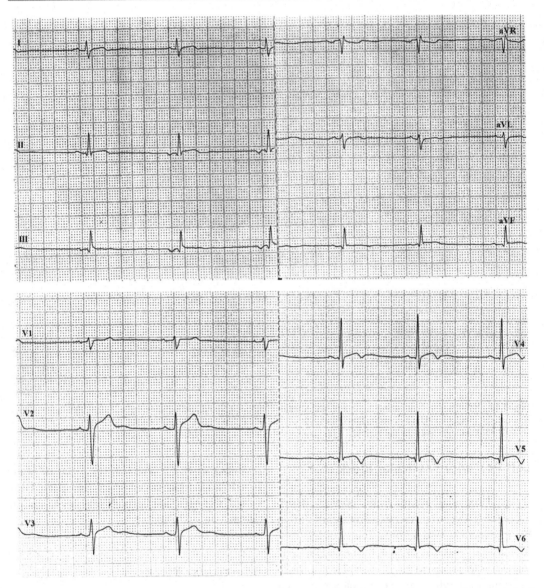

Fig. 8.12 LPFB with axis +90°, RS complex in lead I, qR complexes in leads II and III (with larger R waves in lead III), and small r waves in aVR

The most frequent type involves a RBBB combined with LAFB. It is easy to identify: signs of RBBB (late R waves in lead aVR, S waves in leads V5 and V6) are associated with deviation of the mean QRS axis (past −30°) (Fig. 8.13). The RBBB + left posterior fascicular block (LPFB) pattern is characterized by right axis deviation (+90° and beyond). In these cases, too, it is important to exclude right ventricular hypertrophy as a cause of the axis deviation (Fig. 8.14).

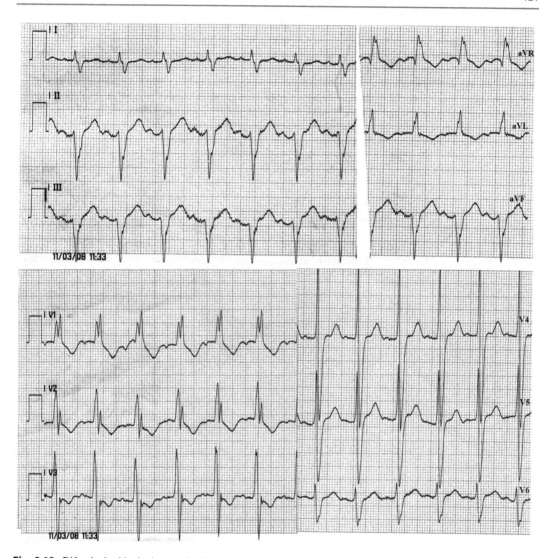

Fig. 8.13 Bifascicular block characterized by complete RBBB, LAFB, and a PR interval of 200 ms

Fig. 8.14 Bifascicular block characterized by RBBB and LPFB. Note the qR complex in V1 and the marked right axis deviation

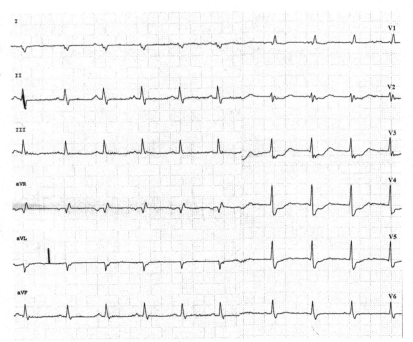

This group of arrhythmias includes several specific syndromes, the most important of which are:

1. The long QT syndrome (LQTS);
2. The short QT syndrome;
3. The Brugada syndrome.

The Long QT Syndrome

The LQTS is a congenital disorder characterized on the surface electrocardiogram (ECG) by abnormal prolongation of the QT interval. The syndrome is caused by genetic mutations that alter the function of transmembrane sodium, potassium, and calcium ion channels, and it is associated with an increased risk of potentially fatal ventricular arrhythmias. The most characteristic is torsade de pointes (TdP)-type ventricular tachycardia (Fig. 6.62), which often causes episodes of syncope but can also lead to sudden death in children and adolescents.

Two main patterns of genetic transmission have been identified. The autosomal recessive form known as the Jervell-Lange Nielsen syndrome is characterized by QT interval prolongation plus deafness. The phenotypic features of the autosomal dominant form (Romano-Ward syndrome) are the same as those of the recessive form without deafness. Over the past decade, at least ten genes have been identified

as causes of LQTS. On the basis of genetic backgrounds, six types of Romano-Ward syndrome and two types of Jervell-Lange Nielsen syndrome are now recognized. Two other rarer forms of LQTS have also been described although not without controversy: LQTS 7 (also known as the Andersen-Tawil syndrome), which is associated with skeletal abnormalities, and the LQTS 8 (or Timothy syndrome), which is associated with congenital heart disease, cognitive problems, and musculoskeletal diseases.

Thus far, ten electrocardiographic types of LQTS have been distinguished, mainly on the basis of the morphology of their T waves. The three most common types (LQTS 1, 2, and 3) are also distinguished by the settings in which the major arrhythmic episodes occur:

1. In LQTS 1, the arrhythmia occurs after physical exertion;
2. in LQTS2, it occurs with emotional stress or at rest;
3. in LQTS3, during sleep or rest.

First-line screening for the LQTS obviously centers on the presence in the ECG of a long QT interval. Durations of <450 ms in males or <460 ms in females are considered normal (Fig. 9.1). It is important to recall that certain commonly used drugs are also capable of prolonging the QT interval. In patients with the LQTS, these drugs can provoke serious

M. Romanò, *Text Atlas of Practical Electrocardiography*,
DOI 10.1007/978-88-470-5741-8_9, © Springer-Verlag Italia 2015

Fig. 9.1 ECG in a patient with the LQTS showing prolongation of the QTc interval (560 ms) and T-U complex (kindly provided by Dr. Carla Giustetto)

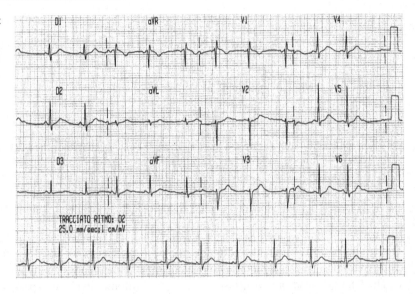

Table 9.1 Drugs and the risk of torsade de pointes (TdP)

1. Drugs that increase the risk of TdP
• Haloperidol
• Amiodarone
• Quinidine
• Disopyramide
• Sotalol
• Procainamide
• Erythromycin
• Clarithromycin
• Thioridazine
• Domperidone
2. Drugs that should be avoided by patients with the LQTS
• Those listed above
• Sibutramine
• Terbutaline
• Sympathomimetic amines (dopamine, dobutamine)
• Phenylephrine
• Cocaine
• Midodrine

ventricular tachyarrhythmias and sometimes sudden death (Table 9.1).

The Short-QT Syndrome

The short-QT syndrome is a recently described clinical entity characterized by an abnormally short QT interval (<300 ms) on the surface ECG, a family history of sudden death, and an increased risk of ventricular fibrillation. Short rate-corrected QT (QTc) intervals are accompanied by morphological changes in the T waves, which are often tall and sharp (Fig. 9.2) or asymmetrical with a normal upslope and an extremely steep downslope.

The risk of arrhythmias is extremely high in patients with the short QT syndrome, in particular ventricular tachyarrhythmias associated with syncope or sudden death. Episodes of atrial fibrillation are also common in these individuals.

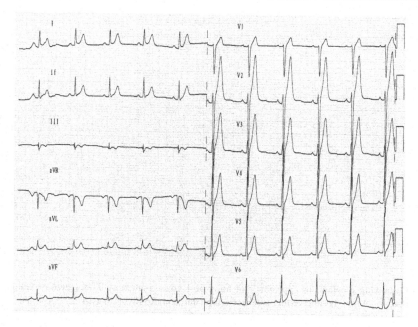

Fig. 9.2 ECG in a patient with the short QT syndrome manifested by a QTc of 280 ms and tall, pointed T waves, especially in the precordial leads (kindly provided by Dr. Carla Giustetto)

The Brugada Syndrome

The Brugada syndrome is a genetic syndrome that was first described in 1992. It is characterized by a high incidence of sudden cardiac death secondary to complex ventricular arrhythmias in young adults whose hearts are structurally sound. The disorder is transmitted in an autosomal dominant manner and is genetically heterogeneous. The mutations responsible for the Brugada syndrome phenotype lead to a reduction in the sodium-ion current that depolarizes the cardiomyocytes. Mutations involving the *SCN5A* gene are found in approximately 20–25% of patients who are clinically diagnosed as having the Brugada syndrome. More recently, the syndrome has also been linked to SCN10A mutation.

Electrocardiographic diagnosis of the disorder is based mainly on the presence of ST-segment elevation in precordial leads V1, V2, and V3, sometimes associated with complete or incomplete right bundle-branch block. The ST-segment elevation includes three main patterns. The type 1 or "coved" pattern is regarded as the most typical, and its appearance under basal conditions or after administration of flecainide or ajmaline is considered diagnostic. The coved pattern consists of a large convex elevation of the ST segment with a J-wave amplitude or ST-segment elevation of ≥2 mm. This is followed (sometimes after a short isoelectric segment) by a negative T wave (Fig. 9.3). The type 2 or "saddle-back" pattern is characterized by a J wave amplitude of ≥2 mm, down-sloping ST-segment elevation (≥1 mm above the

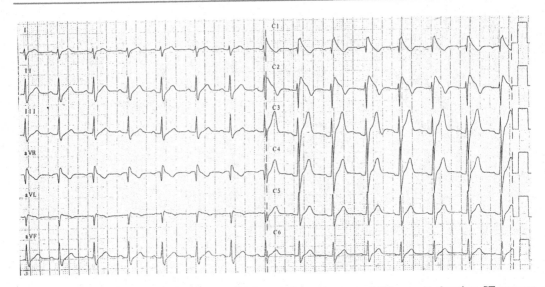

Fig. 9.3 ECG showing spontaneous appearance of the type-1 coved pattern of ST-segment elevation: ST segment convex elevation of >2 mm, no intervening isoelectric segment, and negative T waves

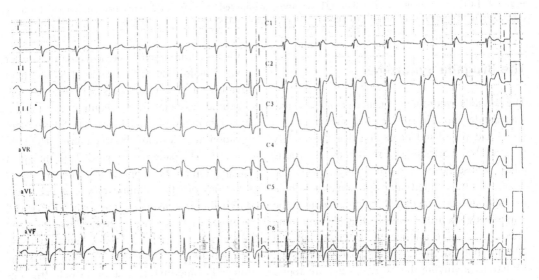

Fig. 9.4 ECG showing the type-2 (saddle-back) pattern of ST-segment elevation: J wave >2 mm followed by down-sloping ST-segment elevation (≥1 mm above the baseline) and positive or biphasic T waves

baseline), and a positive or biphasic T wave (Fig. 9.4). The third type is characterized by mild ST-segment elevation (<1 mm) with the morphologic features of type 1, type 2, or both (Fig. 9.5). Patterns 2 and 3 are suggestive of the Brugada syndrome but not diagnostic unless they

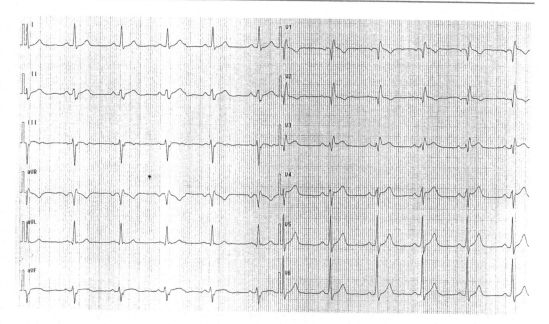

Fig. 9.5 Type 3 pattern of ST-segment elevation characterized by elevation <1 mm and a J wave of ≥2 mm

can be converted to pattern 1 by the administration of sodium channel blockers. The coved and saddleback patterns may appear intermittently. They can be elicited by intravenous infusion of sodium-channel blockers like flecainide, ajmaline, or procainamide (Fig. 9.6).

The arrhythmias usually recorded in patients with the Brugada syndrome are rapid, polymorphic

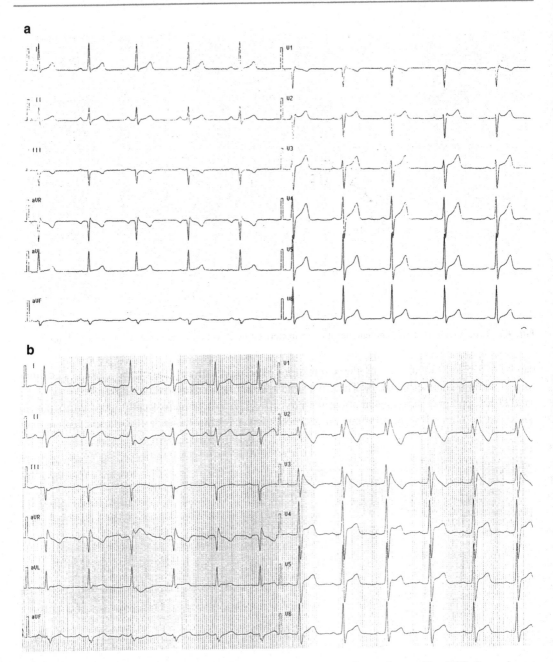

Fig. 9.6 (a) Type-2 ECG pattern suggestive of Brugada syndrome. (b) Intravenous administration of flecainide is followed by conversion to a typical type-1 pattern that is diagnostic of the syndrome. The ECG diagnosis was confirmed by genetic testing

Table 9.2 Drugs that should be avoided by patients with the Brugada syndrome

- Flecainide
- Propafenone
- Procainamide
- Propofol
- Lidocaine
- Bupivacaine
- Cocaine

ventricular tachycardias, ventricular fibrillation, and less commonly monomorphic ventricular tachycardia. The ECG picture typical of the syndrome may appear after a febrile episode or after the administration of drugs (Table 9.2). The similarity between this picture and that of an acute myocardial infarction may complicate electrocardiographic diagnosis of the latter (Fig. 9.7).

Fig. 9.7 (a–c) ECG recorded during an acute septal myocardial infarction: the changes resemble those of the Brugada syndrome

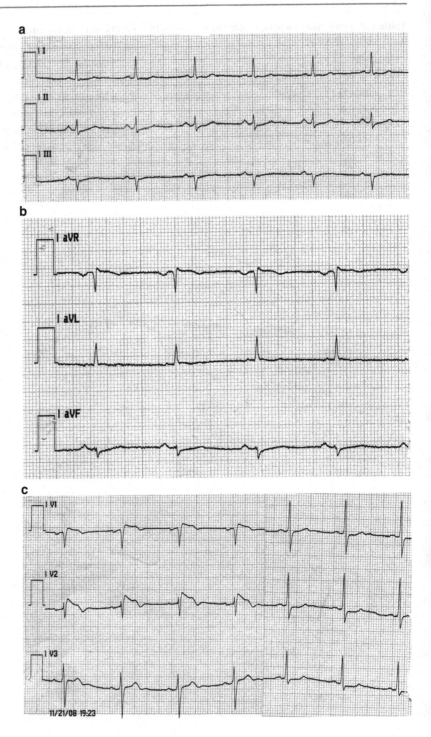

The Electrocardiogram in Patients with Cardiac Pacemakers

10

General Considerations

The heart has the capacity to contract regularly following the delivery of an appropriate electrical stimulus (i.e., adequate in both amplitude and duration) at any point on its surface. In clinical settings, this stimulation is achieved with pacemakers (PM). These devices consist of a pulse generator and one or more leads, which are inserted into the right chamber of the heart (and sometimes the coronary sinus as well) and used to transmit the electrical impulses to the myocardium (Fig. 10.1). The generator is composed of an energy source (lithium battery) and a series of electronic circuits that characterize the PM activity. The leads are attached by screws to a connector block that links them to the generator. Together, they form a "closed" electrical circuit, the dimensions of which vary depending on whether the leads are unipolar or bipolar. In the former case, the circuit consists of an anode (the PM generator) and a cathode (located at the tip of the lead), and it is quite large. For this reason, it is susceptible to interference by external impulses. Bipolar electrodes have two poles at their tips: a proximal one that serves as the anode and a distal one that functions as the cathode. Circuits composed of bipolar electrodes are smaller and much less vulnerable to external interference.

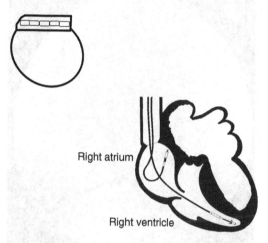

Right atrium

Right ventricle

Fig. 10.1 Schematic showing the positions of the pacemaker leads in the right and left ventricles and their connection to the pulse generator

Pacemakers have two main functions (Table 10.1): *pacing*, which involves stimulation of the myocardium via electrical impulses generated with programmed characteristics (rate, amplitude, and duration); and *sensing*, that is, detection of the heart's own spontaneous electrical activity, expressed in millivolts (amplitude of the intracardiac electrical signal). Detection of electrical activity inhibits the PM, whereas the absence of such signals for a defined period of time (PM timing) reactivates the pacing function. The pacing threshold is the lowest voltage capable of effectively stimulating the

M. Romanò, *Text Atlas of Practical Electrocardiography*,
DOI 10.1007/978-88-470-5741-8_10, © Springer-Verlag Italia 2015

Table 10.1 Key terms related to pacemakers

(a) Pacing: emission of electrical impulses with programmed characteristics (rate, duration in milliseconds, amplitude in volts)

(b) Sensing: detection of spontaneous electrical activity in the heart (intracardiac electric signal)

(c) Pacing threshold: lowest voltage capable of effectively stimulating the myocardial tissue

(d) Sensing threshold: smallest amplitude (in millivolts) of the intracardiac signal that will be detected by the PM sensors

Table 10.2 Main programmable features of pacemakers

(a) Pulse rate (expressed in bpm)

(b) Pulse amplitude (expressed in volts)

(c) Pulse duration (in milliseconds)

(d) Sensitivity (intracardiac signal amplitude—in millivolts—above which PM activity is inhibited)

(e) Atrioventricular delay (in dual-chamber PMs, the time—in milliseconds—that elapses between spontaneous or paced atrial activity and spontaneous or paced ventricular activity)

(f) Lead polarity (unipolar or bipolar)

(g) Ventricular response rate (in rate-responsive PMs—see text)

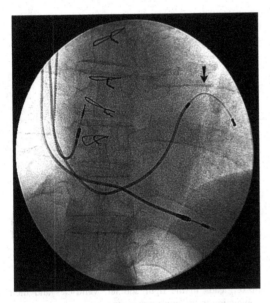

Fig. 10.2 Anteroposterior chest X-ray of the patient with an atriobiventricular pacemaker. The *arrow* indicates the lead placed in the coronary sinus, in the posterolateral branch. The right atrial and right ventricular leads are also visible

myocardial tissue; the sensing threshold is the amplitude of the intracardiac signal.

There are three main types of pacemakers:

1. single-chamber PMs equipped with a single lead inserted in the right atrium or right ventricle;

2. dual-chamber PMs with two leads, one for the right atrium, the other for the right ventricle;

3. triple-chamber or biventricular PMs with three leads, one located in the right atrium, one in the right ventricle, and the third in a cardiac vein, which provides indirect stimulation to the left ventricle as well (Fig. 10.2).

Normal Pacemaker Function

The PMs used today are on-demand models, whose pacing function is activated only when the sensed intrinsic heart rate falls below a certain level, which is programmed for each patient. Table 10.2 shows the other settings that are important in electrocardiographic assessments of PM function. They include the *atrioventricular delay (AVD)* in dual- and triple-chamber PMs (the time that elapses between spontaneous or stimulated activity in the atrium and spontaneous or stimulated activity in the ventricle); *pulse amplitude* and *sensitivity* (intracardiac signal amplitude above which the PM is inhibited). If, for example, the sensitivity is set at 2.5 mV, pacing will be suppressed as long as there are intrinsic electrical signals with amplitudes of >2.5 mV. Lower-amplitude intrinsic signals will not be sensed, and the PM will thus be induced to emit its own electrical impulses.

The pacing rate may be fixed (for example, 70 bpm throughout the day) or variable, a solution aimed at satisfying the changing demands of the organism. Higher rates, for example, are necessary during waking hours and during physical exercise, lower rates when the patient is sleeping. For this reason, PMs are available that "rate-responsive," that is, capable of adjusting the pacing rate in response to changes (detected with special sensors) in muscle activity, oxygen consumption, or other biological parameters. The device can even be programmed to lower the

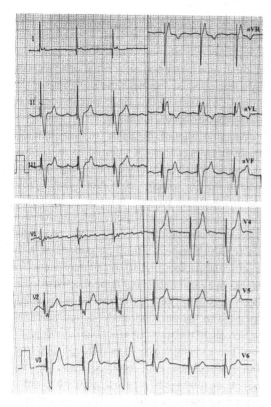

rate during a predefined sleep period (sleep rate). In dual-chamber PMs, an upper tracking rate can also be set, which limits the rate at which the ventricles can be paced in response to intrinsic atrial activity. PM behavior when the upper pacing rate is exceeded varies, depending on the type of arrhythmia and the specific device being used.

The electrocardiographic hallmark of cardiac pacing is an electrical artifact known as a *spike*. It consists of a sharp vertical line, which—in the absence of malfunction—is followed immediately by an atrial or ventricular complex (depending on the site of stimulation). The paced ventricular complex is generally triggered by an impulse generated in the right ventricle, which is therefore activated earlier than the left ventricle. As a result, the QRS complex is broad with a complete LBBB pattern, and it will be positive in lead I and predominantly negative in leads II, III, and aVF (Fig. 10.3). In the presence of atrial pacing, the spike is followed by an atrial depolarization resembling a P wave of sinus origin (Fig. 10.4).

Fig. 10.3 VVI pacing associated with atrial flutter. After every pacing spike, the LBBB-type ventricular complex appears, which is produced by apical stimulation of the right ventricle

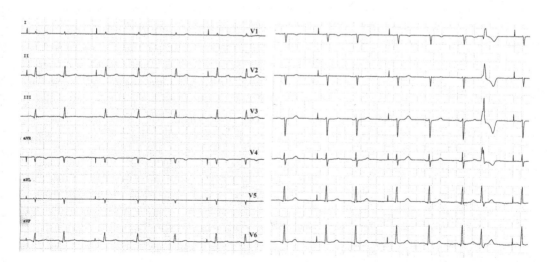

Fig. 10.4 AAI pacing. Sensed sinus activity alternating regularly with pacing spikes followed by P waves that are normally conducted to the ventricles

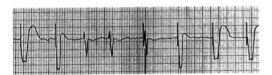

Fig. 10.5 Cardiac monitor strip: The baseline rhythm is atrial fibrillation (AF) with normal conduction to the ventricles (third and fourth complexes). The first and last two complexes are fully paced. The second complex and the third from the end are fusion complexes (with morphologic features midway between those of the spontaneous and paced beats). The fifth complex reflects pseudofusion. The QRS morphology is identical to that of the spontaneous complex: the presence of the spike preceding it is incidental and has no effects

During ventricular pacing, the intrinsic and paced rates are sometimes similar. In this case, the ECG may contained QRS complexes that are completely PM-induced (spike + LBBB-type QRS), those that are completely spontaneous, or *fusion complexes* with an intermediate morphology (spike + incomplete LBBB-type QRS) (Fig. 10.5). The latter are the result of simultaneous activation of the right ventricle by the PM and by impulses generated spontaneously by the heart. Paced beats are also characterized by secondary changes involving ventricular repolarization like those seen in LBBB. *Pseudofusion complexes* may also be recorded: they consist of normal ventricular complexes that are preceded by a pacing spike but have the same rate as the intrinsic rhythm. In this case, depolarization of the ventricles occurs normally.

Mention should be made of a potentially misleading phenomenon referred to as *cardiac memory*, which is induced by long-standing alterations in cardiac activation (e.g., those occurring during pacing). It involves repolarization changes—specifically, pseudoischemic T-wave abnormalities, mainly in the precordial leads, which appear after long periods of right ventricular pacing (Fig. 10.6) and may persist for weeks or even months after normal activation has been restored. They are related to a reversible increase in the duration of the action potential, which alters the transmural repolarization gradient. These changes have to be distinguished from those associated with acute *ischemic* events, which are always difficult to diagnose in patients with permanent pacemakers. They are easier to identify with if the tracing includes both paced and spontaneous complexes.

Fig. 10.6 Upper panel: Tracings recorded by leads V1, V2, and V3 during dual-chamber pacing. Lower panel: Tracings from the same leads in the absence of pacing. Obvious T-wave inversion and QT interval prolongation

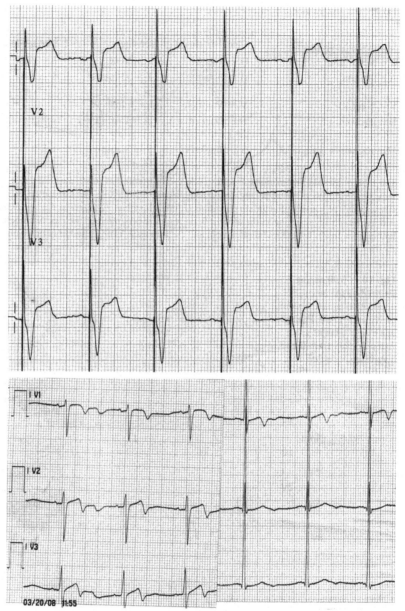

The numerous characteristics and functions of pacemakers are represented by an international code composed of five letters, the first three of which are always expressed (Table 10.3). Various pacing modes can be used:

1. Fixed-rate or *asynchronous pacing* (A00, V00, D00): The sensing circuit is excluded, and the PM emits impulses at a fixed rate, independent of the patient's own rate. This mode has fallen into disuse because of the

Table 10.3 International 5-letter PM code

Chamber paced	Chamber sensed	Response to sensing	Rate modulation	Multisite pacing
0 = None	0 = None	0 = None	0 = None	0 = None
A = Atrium	A = Atrium	T = Triggered	R = Rate modulation	A = Atrium
V = Ventricle	V = Ventricle	I = Inhibited		V = Ventricle
D = Dual (A + V)	D = Dual (A + V)	D = Dual (T + I)		D = Dual (A + V)
Manufacturer's designations only	S = Single (A + V)	S = Single (A + V)		

The table shows the international 5-letter code used to represent functional PM modes. The first and second letters indicate the chambers where pacing and sensing occur, respectively. The third letter indicates the manner in which the PM responds to sensed intracardiac potentials (*I*, inhibit pacing; *T*, triggered pacing; *D*, inhibit pacing in the ventricle and inhibit or trigger pacing in the atrium; *0*, no response programmed, i.e., asynchronous). The fourth letter indicates both programmability and rate modulation, and the fifth letter is now used to indicate multisite pacing, when indicated

Fig. 10.7 V00 pacing induced by magnet application and exclusion of sensing circuit. Pacing spikes are generated independently from the spontaneous rhythm

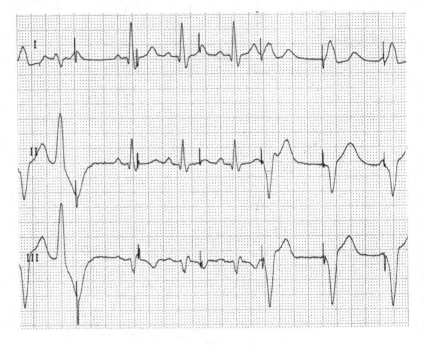

risks associated with its interference with the patient's intrinsic rhythm. However, it can sometimes activated temporarily (by passing a magnet over the pacemaker) to assess the pulse efficacy when pacing is being inhibited by the patient's rhythm (Fig. 10.7).

2. *On-demand* or inhibited pacing (AAI, VVI): This is the most widely used mode because it respects the patient's intrinsic rhythm. Detection of electrical activity inhibits the emission of PM impulses; stimulation is reactivated by the absence of recorded activity for a certain period of time (PM timing, a programmable parameter) (Figs. 10.3 and 10.4).

3. Ventricular pacing with *atrial tracking* (VDD): The ventricular impulse is synchronized with the spontaneous atrial activity of the patient. Each intrinsic P wave is followed (after a preset AVD) by the delivery of a ventricular pulse. This mode of pacing is achieved with a special lead, which is placed in the apex of the right ventricle and has a dipole located in its

Fig. 10.8 VDD pacing. Limb leads: Each spontaneously generated P wave is followed, after a constant AVD, by a paced ventricular complex

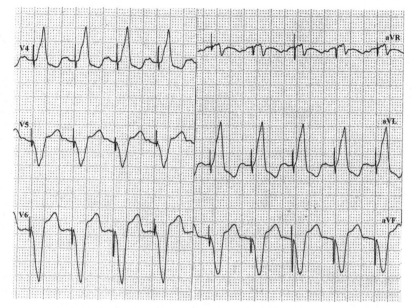

Fig. 10.9 VVIR pacing. The baseline rate is set at 70 bpm. In this tracing it increases to 100 bpm during physical activity

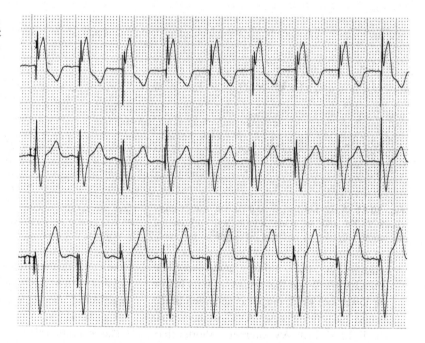

proximal segment, which will be located in the right atrium. The dipole is capable of sensing spontaneous sinus depolarizations but it cannot pace the atria. VDD pacing is useful in patients with advanced AV blocks and preserved sinus node function (Fig. 10.8).

4. *Rate-responsive* pacing (AAIR, VVIR, DDDR): compared with the single pacing modes, the only difference is the rate of stimulation (Fig. 10.9).

5. *Dual-chamber* pacing (DDD) requires insertion of two leads, which allow pacing and

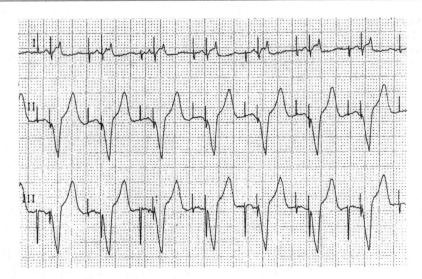

Fig. 10.10 DDD pacing. Two pacing artifacts can be seen: one generated in the right atrium and followed by a P wave; the second generated in the right ventricle and followed by an LBBB-type ventricular complex

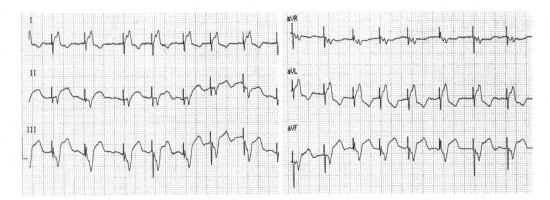

Fig. 10.11 Atrial fibrillation in a patient with a dual-chamber PM and an acute inferior-wall myocardial infarction reflected by inferior ST-segment elevation. There are no discernible P waves, and the ventricular rate is approximately 110 bpm. Note the irregular rate of the ventricular spikes

sensing in the atrium and ventricle (Fig. 10.10). When the sinus rate falls below the lower rate limit, output is activated in the atrium and, after a preset AVD, in the ventricle. If the intrinsic AV interval is shorter than the programmed AVD, the atrial wave will be followed by normal ventricular depolarization. If the sinus rate exceeds the programmed rate and the intrinsic AV interval exceeds the programmed AVD, VDD pacing will be activated (see above). The onset of AF in a patient with a dual-chamber PM deserves special attention: the high atrial rates in this case can "drag" the ventricular pacing rate upward (Fig. 10.11).

The pacing artifacts shown in the figures presented thus far are associated with unipolar pacing (see above). They are appreciably different from those seen during bipolar stimulation: the reduced dimensions of the circuit in this case result in a low-amplitude spike, which is not always easy to identify (Figs. 10.12 and 10.13).

Fig. 10.12 Bipolar AAI pacing with a long P-V interval due to slow atrioventricular conduction. Pacing artifact (*arrow*)

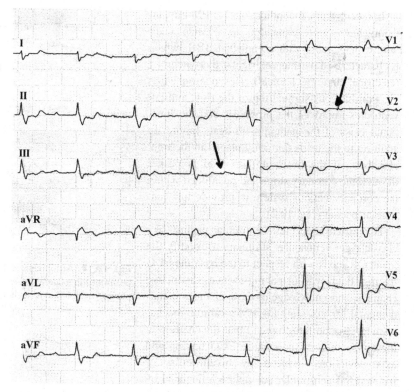

Fig. 10.13 Bipolar DDD pacing: *arrows* indicate the presence of atrial and ventricular pacing artifacts

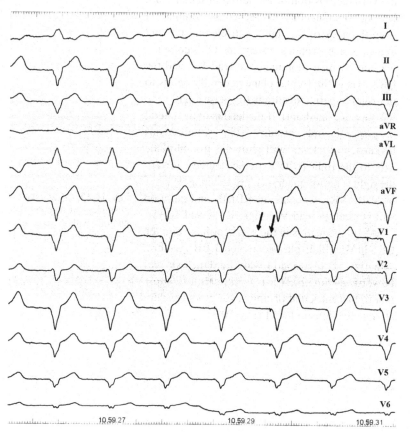

In recent years, the indications for PM implantation have been expanded to include heart failure in patients with complete LBBB, which is characterized by interventricular dyssynchrony (electrical and mechanical). Resynchronization via simultaneous stimulation of the right and left ventricles improves the prognosis and the functional class of the patient with heart failure. In addition to the leads normally placed in the right chambers of the heart, a third lead is passed through the coronary sinus and positioned within the coronary venous system to provide left ventricular pacing (Fig. 10.2).

Biventricular and left ventricular pacing (like classic right ventricular stimulation) modify the mean QRS axis with respect to the baseline ECG tracing. Each type of pacing induces distinctive changes, and knowledge of these changes is fundamental for assessing the PM's capture mechanism. It is important to recall that the changes in the appearance of the surface ECG tracing and axis deviations induced by biventricular or isolated left ventricular pacing are influenced by the variable position of the left-ventricular lead. During simultaneous biventricular stimulation from the apex of the right ventricle and LV site in the coronary venous system, the QRS complex is often positive (dominant) in lead V1, and the QRS axis in the frontal plane generally points to the right superior quadrant (or occasionally the left superior quadrant). If the lead is in the lateral or posterolateral coronary vein, simultaneous biventricular pacing will shift the frontal-plane axis to the right (with extreme degrees, toward the right superior quadrant) (predominant R wave in lead aVR), whereas an RBBB configuration will be seen in lead V1 (Figs. 10.14 and 10.15). If instead the lead is in the great cardiac vein, the QRS in V1 will display a complete LBBB pattern, sometimes with a small r wave, and the axis will be vertical (Fig. 10.16). It is important to stress that right-ventricular pacing never produces negative deflections in lead I (Fig. 10.3).

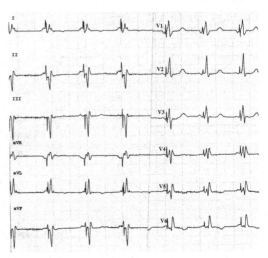

Fig. 10.14 Atriobiventricular pacing with the left lead positioned in a lateral branch. Complete RBBB-type morphology with left axis deviation. Limb leads are shown on the *left*; precordial leads on the *right*

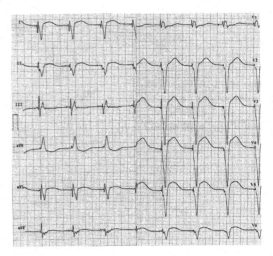

Fig. 10.15 Atriobiventricular pacing with the left lead positioned in a posterolateral branch. RBBB-type morphology with extreme left axis deviation. Limb leads are shown on the *left*; precordial leads on the *right*

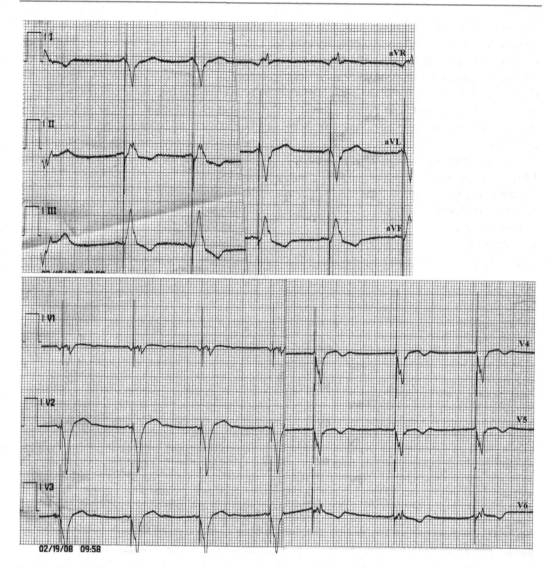

Fig. 10.16 Atriobiventricular pacing with the left lead positioned in the great cardiac vein: LBBB-type morphology with vertical axis

After the leads are placed in the cardiac chambers, they undergo a process of *maturation*. Trauma to the cells at the implantation site causes edema and the development of a fibrotic capsule around the tip of the electrode. The presence of this nonexcitable scar tissue increases the amount of energy required to capture the ventricle. Therefore, the pacing threshold rises progressively, reaching a peak 2–3 weeks after implantation. Thereafter, it tends to decrease somewhat and remain stable. These changes have to be considered during investigation of possible PM malfunction because in some cases, the threshold increase is large enough to impair pacing.

Pacemaker Malfunction

Pacemaker malfunction can be caused by problems involving the pulse generator or leads or by patient-level factors (e.g., acute ischemia, antiarrhythmic drug therapy) that affect the pacing or sensing thresholds. It is also important to recall that in some cases, the malfunction is only apparent (pseudo-malfunction): the device is actually functioning normally. To properly evaluate the ECG of a patient with a PM, one should have access to certain information, which is not always available. It includes the pacing mode and rate, pulse amplitude and duration, sensitivity, and any special algorithms that have been activated.

PM malfunctions can be divided into the following categories:

1. Failure to pace;
2. failure to capture;
3. undersensing;
4. oversensing.

Failure to Pace

This type of malfunction is characterized by the absence of an impulse capable of capturing the myocardium. The impulse is emitted by the generator but is not transferred to the electrode. Failure to pace can be caused by:

- faulty connection between the stimulating electrode and the pulse generator (loose set screws);
- lead malfunction;
- battery depletion;
- circuit malfunction.

The ECG is characterized by the absence of pacing spikes and a rate below the programmed lower rate limit (Fig. 10.17).

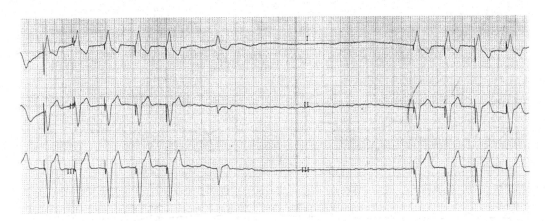

Fig. 10.17 Prolonged, transient PM failure to pace: absence of the ventricular pacing spike is followed by asystole

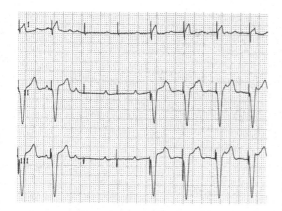

Fig. 10.18 Intermittent failure to capture in a patient with complete AVB and a VVI PM: two nonconducted spikes are seen which result in asystole

Failure to Capture

In this case, the pacing spike is visible on ECG, but it is not followed by an atrial or ventricular depolarization. The various causes of this type of malfunction include:

- an increase in the pacing threshold (electrode maturation);
- dislodgment of the leads;
- perforation of the myocardium;
- defective lead insulation;
- lead fracture;
- faulty connection between the stimulating electrode and the generator (loose set screws);
- battery depletion;

- myocardial infarction;
- antiarrhythmic drug therapy;
- exit block.

The surface ECG in this case will be characterized by absence of depolarization after the spike (Fig. 10.18).

Undersensing

Undersensing is the failure of the PM to properly detect native electrical activity and inhibit pacing when it is present. As a result, impulse delivery by the generator occurs inappropriately. The causes of undersensing include:

- inappropriate sensitivity setting;
- lead dislodgement;
- defective lead insulation;
- fractured lead;
- battery depletion;
- electrode maturation, which increases the pacing threshold and reduces the amplitude of the intracardiac signal detected by the PM;
- myocardial infarction;
- electrolyte abnormalities;
- asynchronous pacing mode (see above).

An ECG recorded during undersensing shows intrinsic atrial and/or ventricular depolarization that is not detected by the PM and the emission of atrial and/or ventricular pacing spikes that are independent from the spontaneous rhythm (competing rhythm) (Fig. 10.19).

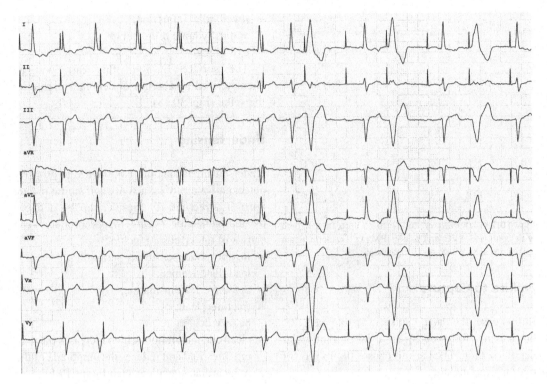

Fig. 10.19 Failure to sense in a patient with a VVI PM. Pacing spikes, independent from spontaneous electrical activity, fall on the T waves, sometimes eliciting a premature R-on-T complex capable of triggering malignant ventricular arrhythmias. Intermittent failure to capture is also seen. Typical signs of a dislodged PM lead

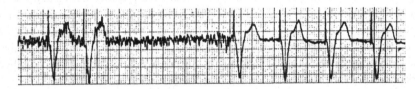

Fig. 10.20 Myopotential oversensing (detection of pectoral muscle contractions that inhibits pacing) in a patient with VVIR PM

Oversensing

This type of malfunction involves inappropriate inhibition of PM output prompted by sensing of a nonphysiological electrical signal. In PM-dependent patients or those with extremely slow spontaneous rates, oversensing can cause life-threatening episodes of asystole or bradycardia (Fig. 10.20). The causes of oversensing include:

– lead fracture;
– defective lead insulation;
– myopotential inhibition (i.e., inhibition produced by sensed skeletal muscle contractions—the most common cause);
– electromagnetic interference from an external source;
– inappropriate sensitivity setting;
– faulty connection between the stimulating electrode and the generator (loose set screws);
– very high-amplitude T waves that are mistakenly sensed as QRS complexes.

Pseudomalfunction

Sometimes the ECG features seem to be suggestive of PM malfunction when the device is actually

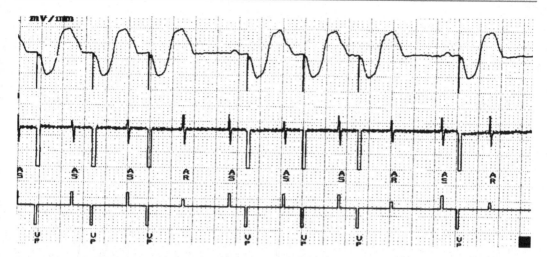

Fig. 10.21 ECG telemetry strip from a patient with a DDD PM and atrial tachycardia. The Wenckebach-type protective mechanism is reflected by intermittent lengthening of the programmed AVD and the equally intermittent absence of ventricular pacing output. Top tracing: surface ECG recording; middle tracing: intraatrial recording showing electrical activity in the atria; bottom tracing: marker channels. *AS*, atrial sensing; *VP*, ventricular pacing

working properly. These pseudomalfunctions can be related to:

1. changes in the ECG morphology;
2. changes in the pacing rate;
3. changes in the AVD or refractory periods.

1. When the paced and spontaneous rates are similar, one sometimes sees a QRS complex that is preceded by a pacing spike but shaped like spontaneous complex. These *pseudofusion complexes* (Fig. 10.5) are normal and must be distinguished from signs of PM malfunction.
2. Changes in the pacing rate can occur during several situations characterized by normal PM operation. They include:
   - magnet-activation of the asynchronous pacing mode at a rate other than that programmed (Fig. 10.6).
   - rates above the programmed upper rate limit. In this case, different PM behaviors may be seen, all aimed mainly at limiting the rate increase that would occur in the presence of atrial tachycardia (Fig. 10.21).
   - electrical resetting caused by electromagnetic interference from external sources (electrosurgical devices, defibrillation, etc.). The PM response varies, but in general it involves conversion to asynchronous pacing (V00 or D00).

   - battery depletion (heralded by rate decreases).
   - PM-mediated tachycardia (a peculiar form of supraventricular tachycardia typically associated with pacing modes that allow detection of intrinsic atrial activity i.e., DDD or single-lead VDD pacing). In patients with normal atrioventricular conduction, a premature ventricular beat may be retro-conducted to the atria. If it arrives after the atrial refractory period has ended, it will be sensed and conducted to the ventricles after the programmed AVD. The paced ventricular beat is then re-conducted back to the atria, giving rise to a reentrant tachycardia with a rate that is close to the programmed upper rate limit (Fig. 10.22).
   - Programming in rate-responsive mode (Fig. 10.8).

3. Safety pacing is designed to provide pacing support when needed. However, it may also be activated in the presence of atrial undersensing. For example, if a P wave is not sensed (for any of the reasons listed above), the pacemaker emits an atrial impulse followed shortly thereafter by a ventricular impulse (Fig. 10.23).

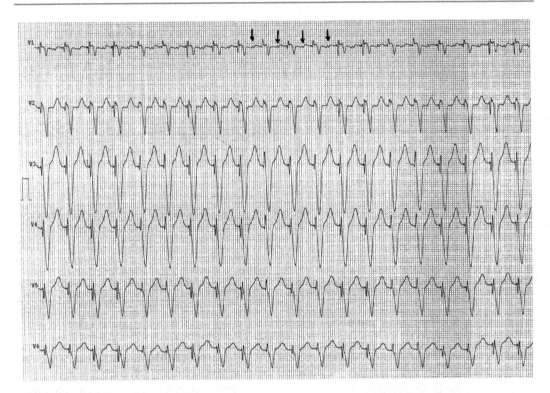

Fig. 10.22 PM-mediated tachycardia. The *arrows* indicate retro-conducted P waves; the QRS complexes are preceded by obvious pacing spikes

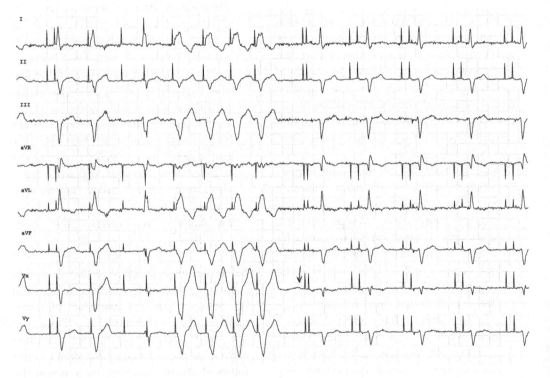

Fig. 10.23 Safety pacing. The *arrow* indicates the sensing defect, which prompts atrioventricular pacing output with a PV interval shorter than that programmed, as shown by the rest of the tracing

The Electrocardiogram in Ischemic Heart Disease

11

General Considerations

Reductions in blood flow (and consequently the oxygen supply) to the myocardium can cause transient or permanent damage (ischemia and necrosis, respectively). Atherosclerosis of the coronary arteries is the most common cause. In most cases, the ischemia initially involves the subendocardial layers of the myocardium, which are characterized by a higher metabolic rate and oxygen consumption than the subepicardial layers since they more exposed to extravascular compressive forces (systolic tension, ventricular filling pressure). Only later does the

damage extends to the full thickness of the myocardium (Fig. 11.1).

The main electrocardiographic (ECG) changes associated with myocardial ischemia involve the ST segment, the T wave, and the QRS complex. The nature and time-courses of these changes vary depending on the extension and temporal characteristics (acute vs. chronic, transient vs. persistent) of the ischemia and on the concomitant presence of other factors that can complicate diagnosis (bundle-branch blocks, pacemaker rhythms, WPW-type ventricular preexcitation).

Acute ischemia modifies the morphology and duration of the transmembrane action potential of the myocardial cells. Those of the subendocardial layers display decreases in the resting potential, the amplitude and velocity of phase 0, and the duration of the action potential (Fig. 11.2a). The result is an electrical gradient between ischemic and normal cells during the whole cardiac cycle. The ischemia may be caused by incomplete occlusion of a coronary vessel, in which case it will be confined to the inner layers of the myocardium (subendocardial ischemia), or by complete (transient or permanent) occlusion, in which case it will involve the full thickness of the myocardium (transmural ischemia).

The main ECG correlate of acute ischemia is displacement of the ST-segment from its normal

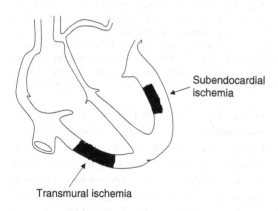

Subendocardial ischemia

Transmural ischemia

Fig. 11.1 Schematic comparison of transmural ischemia from that confined to the subendocardial layers. See text for details

M. Romanò, *Text Atlas of Practical Electrocardiography*,
DOI 10.1007/978-88-470-5741-8_11, © Springer-Verlag Italia 2015

a

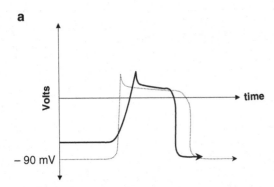

b

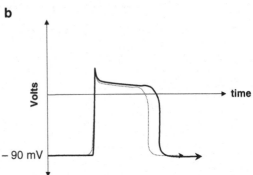

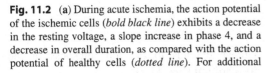

Fig. 11.2 (**a**) During acute ischemia, the action potential of the ischemic cells (*bold black line*) exhibits a decrease in the resting voltage, a slope increase in phase 4, and a decrease in overall duration, as compared with the action potential of healthy cells (*dotted line*). For additional details, see Chap. 1. (**b**) During chronic ischemia, the action potential of the ischemic cells (*bold black line*) displays an increase in duration with respect to that of healthy cells (*dotted line*)

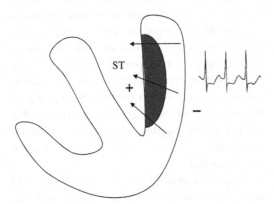

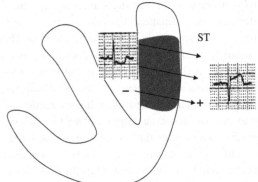

Fig. 11.3 In subendocardial ischemia, the electrical vector is moving away from the healthy area of the myocardium (electronegative) and toward the ischemic zone (electrically positive). The leads facing the latter zone will thus record a depression of the ST segment

Fig. 11.4 During transmural ischemia, the electrical vector is directed from the electronegative endocardium to the electropositive epicardium. The overlying lead records an approaching vector—therefore an elevation of the ST segment—while the lead exploring the opposite wall records a vector moving away from it, which will be reflected by reciprocal depression of the ST segment

position on the isoelectric line, which reflects the tendency of normal cardiomyocytes to repolarize in a uniform manner. In the presence of subendocardial ischemia, the leads "facing" the affected area record a depressed ST segment (Fig. 11.3). In contrast, transmural ischemia will be associated with ST-segment elevation in these leads and reciprocal ST-segment depression in the leads whose positive poles are oppositely directed (Fig. 11.4). Transmural ischemia can also produce significant changes in the T waves with the same electrical and clinical implications. The initial phase of ischemia is associated with an increase in voltage (T-wave peaking, referred to as hyperacute T-wave changes). It may be followed by ST-segment elevation and T-wave pseudonormalization (positivity of T waves that are negative under baseline conditions). Unlike the ECG changes that occur during subendocardial ischemia, those associated with transmural ischemia are closely correlated with the affected region of the myocardium.

Two different mechanisms have been proposed to explain ischemic elevation of the ST segment. The first assumes that the elevation is produced during *electrical diastole*, the ECG correlate of which is the TQ interval. In this case, the elevation is believed to reflect partial or complete depolarization of the ischemic cells, whose electrical charge is negative relative to their nonischemic counterparts, during phase 4 of the action potential. The result would be a flow of current (the so-called current of injury) represented by a vector directed away from the ischemic zone toward the nonischemic areas, which are positively charged during diastole. On ECG, these events would translate into TQ-segment *depression* (Fig. 11.5a) in the leads facing the ischemic zone. However, the electrocardiographs commonly used in clinical settings, which operate on AC power, automatically realign the TQ segment with the isoelectric line, thereby producing an *apparent* level change in the ST-segment, which is equal in magnitude and opposite in direction to the level change involving the TQ segment.

The second hypothesis assumes that the current of injury develops during *electrical systole* (Fig. 11.5b), which corresponds to the ST segment itself. It is based on the electrophysiological alterations in ischemic cells mentioned above (i.e., reduction of the resting potential, reduction of the amplitude and velocity of phase 0, and reduction of the overall duration of the action potential). These conditions result in an electrical current that flows from the nonischemic zone (where the cells are normally depolarized and therefore electronegative) toward the ischemic zone, which is prematurely repolarized or incompletely depolarized. The leads over the ischemic zone therefore record an elevation of the ST segment, which, as noted earlier, is often associated with reciprocal ST-segment depression in the opposite leads.

The phenomenon of ST-segment depression is caused mainly by delayed repolarization phase in the ischemic subendocardial zone. The ST-segment vector is therefore directed as usual from the epicardial to the endocardial layers, that is, from the nonischemic to the ischemic zone

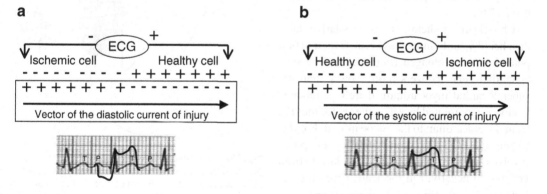

ST-segment changes and the current of injury ECG

a

b

Fig. 11.5 ST-segment changes in the diastolic (**a**) and systolic (**b**) current of injury hypotheses. See text for details

Fig. 11.6 Holter
recording from a patient
experiencing episodes of
subendocardial ischemia.
Top strip (baseline
conditions): Mild (<1 mm)
ST-segment depression.
Middle strip: The
depression (horizontal)
becomes more marked
(4 mm). Bottom strip: As
the ischemia becomes more
severe, the morphology of
the ST segment changes
again: the down-sloping
depression is a peculiar,
specific characteristic of
myocardial ischemia

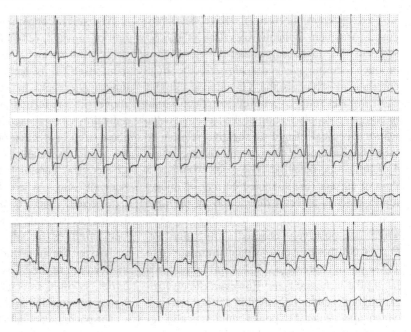

(Fig. 11.3). ST-segment depression is often
associated with prolongation of the QT interval.
The shape and appearance of the depressed ST
segment is important: horizontal and down-
sloping ST depressions of at least 1 mm are
considered significant, whereas the significance
threshold for up-sloping depressions is 1.5 mm
(Fig. 11.6).

Chronically ischemic cells repolarize later
than healthy cardiomyocytes because their action
potentials are prolonged (Fig. 11.2b). The subepicardial zone recovers more slowly than the
subendocardial myocardium: therefore, repolarization is represented by a T-wave vector moving
from the epicardium to the endocardium. For this
reason, the ECG alteration typical of this phase
involves an inversion of T-wave polarity (from
positive to negative) in the leads exploring the
ischemic region (Fig. 11.7). Under these conditions, T-wave negativity in a given lead is

generally associated with transmural ischemia
in the area being explored by that lead.

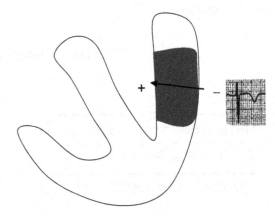

Fig. 11.7 Schematic of the T-wave vector in the chronic
phase of transmural ischemia: the subepicardial area is
electronegative since it repolarizes later than the
subendocardial area. The vector moves away from the
exploring electrode and a negative T wave is recorded

The QRS-complex changes classically associated with myocardial necrosis appear in the post-acute phase of infarction and consist of "new" Q waves (not seen on previous recordings) with a duration of ≥40 ms and an amplitude at least one fourth that of the R wave in the same lead. It is important to recall that, in certain leads (the precordials in particular), Q waves can be physiological, reflecting septal depolarization. Pathologic Q waves will be found in two or more anatomically contiguous leads. This is especially true of lead III, where the appearance of Q waves is considered abnormal only if they are also present in leads II and aVF.

Q waves are a reflection of the necrotic tissue's electrical inertness, that is, its inability to generate the electrical activity that would normally counterbalance similar forces originating in the opposite wall. The absence of electrical activity in a specific area results in the appearance of a QRS vector moving away from the necrotic zone and therefore inscribed as a negative deflection (Fig. 11.8). Abnormal Q waves were once considered a distinguishing feature of transmural myocardial infarctions. It has now become clear, however, that they may also develop in patients with nontransmural necrosis. Even more important, Q waves may well be absent in cases of transmural necrosis. As a result, myocardial infarctions are now electrocardiographically classified as Q-wave or non-Q-wave MIs. In the latter cases, the ECG alterations are confined to the ST segment and T wave. Phases of transient ischemia may also be associated with QRS alterations, mainly consisting of increased in amplitude and conduction disturbances. (Examples will be provided below in the section on angioplasty.)

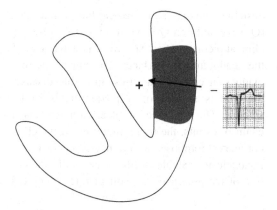

Fig. 11.8 QRS vector in the presence of necrosis: the vector is moving away from the electrode, so a negative deflection (Q wave) is recorded

It is important to stress that the ST-segment and T-wave changes that develop during ischemic heart disease (T-wave inversion in particular) may also appear in nonischemic forms of heart disease (left ventricular overload, myocarditis, pericarditis, hypertrophic cardiomyopathy), during certain types of drug therapy or electrolyte imbalances, and even in young persons (females in particular) with no significant heart disease. The saying that an ECG must first be described and then interpreted is never so true as in ischemic heart disease, and it becomes a valid basis for diagnosis only when analyzed within the specific clinical context of the case at hand. Failure to recall this rule can lead to misdiagnosis, sometimes with grave consequences.

Clinical and Electrocardiographic Pictures

The main clinical manifestations of coronary heart disease are stable angina pectoris and the acute coronary syndromes, which include unstable angina and myocardial infarctions (Q-wave and non-Q-wave forms). The different clinical pictures reflect specific characteristics of the endoluminal surfaces of atherosclerotic plaques in coronary arteries. In stable disease, the fibrous surface of a plaque tends to be smooth. The presence of ulceration triggers a chain of events, the most important of which is coronary thrombosis, which may be occlusive or nonocclusive. Stable angina is generally indicative of the presence of a soft plaque. Ulcerated plaques with thrombosis may be associated with myocardial infarction or unstable angina.

Stable Angina Pectoris

In patients with stable angina, the ischemic episodes are usually associated with sub-endocardial ischemia, which is expressed on the ECG by ST-segment depression that varies in magnitude and extension with the extension of the coronary artery disease (Fig. 11.9).

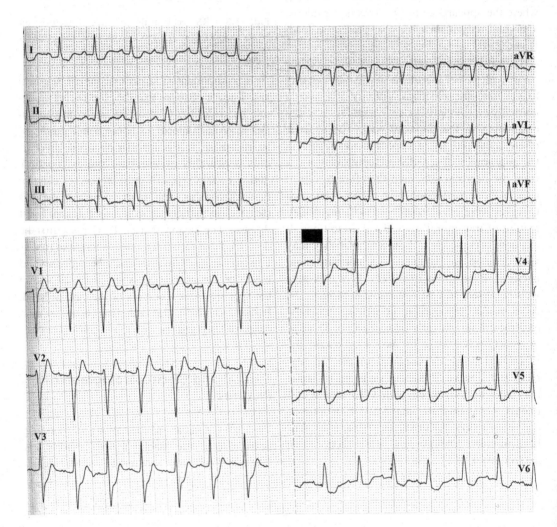

Fig. 11.9 Subendocardial ischemia associated with exertional angina in a patient will multivessel disease involving the left main coronary artery and the right coronary artery. A lesion of the latter was responsible for the prior inferior myocardial infarction reflected by the small Q waves in the inferior leads. The remarkable extension of the coronary artery disease is reflected by the magnitude of the ST-segment depression and the number of leads in which it appears (leads V2 through V6, I, and aVL). Limb leads are shown at the *top*, precordial leads at the *bottom*

During the ischemia-free intervals the ECG returns to its baseline pattern, which is often normal. Ischemia develops when oxygen consumption increases as a result of physical exertion, a hypertensive crisis, anemia, emotional stress, etc. In rare cases, ECGs recorded during angina secondary to subocclusive coronary lesions will display ST-segment elevation or transient positivity of T waves that were formerly negative.

Unstable Angina

In this case, the ischemia is recurrent and no longer confined to periods of increased oxygen consumption, occurring also at rest. The ECG changes range from ST-segment depression (reflecting subendocardial ischemia) (Fig. 11.8) to ST-segment elevation (Fig. 11.10) or pseudo-normalization of T waves (Fig. 11.11). In recent years, greater emphasis has been placed on the

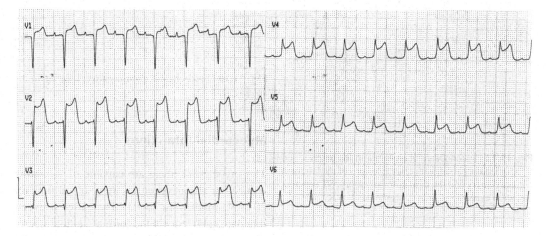

Fig. 11.10 Precordial lead tracings from a patient with unstable angina and transient ST-segment elevation caused by critical lesion of the proximal LAD

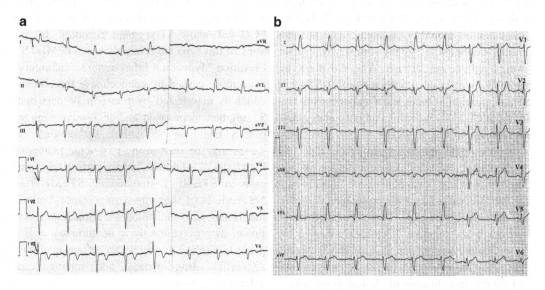

Fig. 11.11 Transmural ischemia during an episode of unstable angina secondary to critical stenosis of the left anterior descending artery. The ischemic area extends beyond the apex and involves part of the inferior wall.

The baseline ECG (**a**) shows negative T waves in the anterior and inferior leads. During ischemia (**b**) the T waves in these leads become positive

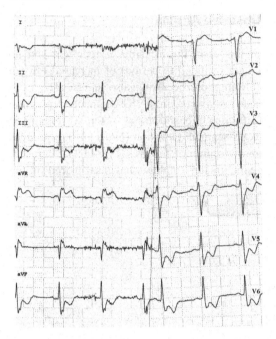

Fig. 11.12 Subendocardial ischemia in the anterior and inferior leads a patient with critical lesions of the left main coronary artery and the right coronary artery. ST-segment elevation exceeding 2 mm is seen in lead aVR

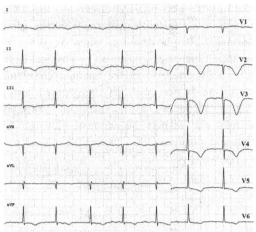

Fig. 11.13 Postischemic giant negative T waves in the anterior leads

Myocardial Infarctions

The myocardial fibers are capable of tolerating reduced or absent coronary artery blood flow for 20 or 30 minutes (ischemia). Thereafter, irreversible damage occurs in the form of cellular necrosis. Acute myocardial infarctions are customarily divided into two categories based on the nature of the coronary artery thrombosis. In the presence of occlusive thrombosis, the acute-phase ECG will show ST-segment elevation. Infarctions of this type are referred to as STEMIs (ST Elevation Myocardial Infarctions) to distinguish from those caused by nonocclusive thrombosis, which is manifested by transient or persistent ST-segment depression and/or T-wave changes (non-STEMIs or NSTEMIs). Pathological Q-waves may be seen in the post-acute phases of both types of infarction, but are particularly common in STEMI. Distinguishing STEMI from NSTEMI is of the utmost importance because the former is an indication for immediate reperfusion therapy (fibrinolysis or coronary angioplasty), whereas the latter can be managed with aggressive drug therapy and interventional solutions deferred.

role of lead aVR in assessments of the extension of coronary artery disease. ST-segment elevation in this lead has in fact been strongly linked to high rates of mortality, ischemic events, and critical lesions of left main coronary artery or severe triple-vessel disease. The elevation in lead aVR is associated with reciprocal ST-segment depression in other leads and is considered an important ECG index of coronary artery disease extension (Fig. 11.12).

After several hours to several days of repeated or protracted episodes of ischemia, it is not uncommon to see T-wave inversion in leads facing the affected zone, with prolongation of the QT interval (Fig. 11.13). These so-called post-ischemic giant negative T waves are caused by the prolonged action potential of the ischemic cells: they are unrelated to the acute ischemia and are not an indication of clinical worsening.

Non-ST-Elevation Myocardial Infarction

The ECG changes seen in the initial phases of an NSTEMI involve the ST segment and T waves and resemble those described above for unstable angina. In rare cases, NSTEMIs may be associated with transient ST-segment elevation, which reflects temporary aggravation of the non-occlusive thrombosis by superimposed spasm of the affected coronary artery and is not followed by the development of Q waves.

ST-Elevation Myocardial Infarction

The main ECG alterations observed in patients with STEMIs include ST-segment elevation in the leads facing the ischemic area, followed by T-wave inversion and the appearance of new Q waves. In the initial phases of the MI, tall, peaked T waves may be recorded as a reflection of transmural ischemia. In the chronic phases, the ST-segment elevation tends to disappear. Much later, the negative T waves may also become positive again, leaving the Q wave as the only ECG sign of the infarction (Fig. 11.14).

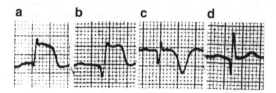

Fig. 11.14 ECG changes in the various phases of myocardial infarction. (**a**) Stage 1: ST-segment elevation; (**b**) Stage 2. Appearance of Q waves; (**c**) Stage 3. ST segment isoelectricity restored and T-wave inversion; (**d**) Stage 4 (rare). Normalization of T-wave polarity, leaving the Q-wave as the only remaining sign of MI

As noted above, the ST-segment and QRS changes are sensitive, specific predictors of the areas affected by the ischemia and necrosis and of the coronary artery that is occluded (Table 11.1). The locations of the coronary arteries are shown in Fig. 11.15, and the diagram in Fig. 11.16 summarizes the distribution of coronary artery blood flow to the various segments of the left ventricle (as defined by the American Heart Association). Figure 11.17 shows the correlation between coronary anatomy, perfusion of the myocardial segments, and ECG localization of ST-segment and QRS alterations.

It is important to note that studies correlating ECG signs of necrosis with magnetic resonance findings have shown that, in contrast with traditional views, the position of the heart within the chest cavity reveals the limited importance of the so-called posterior wall. The longitudinal vertical plane is not precisely sagittal, relative to the anteroposterior position, but rather oblique and directed toward the left. It follows then that the portion of the heart formerly considered posterior, relative to the precordial leads V1-V3, is actually lateral. Therefore, from an electrocardiographic point of view, the posterior wall seems irrelevant: what for years has been defined as a posterior infarction (tall R waves in V1-V2) is actually located in the lateral wall. The terminology used in this book is that proposed in 2006 by Bayes de Luna.

Table 11.1 Correlation between ECG patterns, infarcted myocardial segments, and culprit coronary vessel. (Modified from Bayes de Luna et al., 2006)

Name	ECG pattern	Infarcted segments	Occlusion site
Septal	QS in V1-V2	2–8	LAD with S1
Apical-anterior	QS in V1→V6	7, 8, 13, 14, 17	LAD distal to S1-D1
Extensive anterior	QS in V1→V6, I aVL	1, 2, 4, 7, 8, 13, 14, 17	Proximal LAD
Mid-anterior	QS in aVL, I, V2-V3	1, 7, 13	D1
Lateral	Q in I, aVL, RS V1-V2	5, 6, 11, 12	OM, LCx or INT
Inferior	Q in II, III, and aVF	4, 10, 15	RCA, LCx
Inferolateral	Q in II, III, aVF, I, aVL and/or RS V1-V2	4, 5, 10, 11, 15	Dominant RCA or LCx

LCx, left circumflex artery; *RCA*, right coronary artery; *D1*, first diagonal branch; *OM*, obtuse marginal branch; *INT*, intermediate branch; *S1*, first septal branch; *LAD*, left anterior descending artery

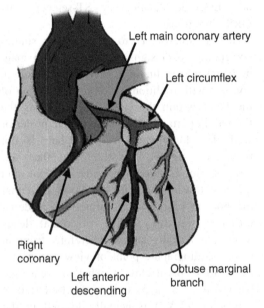

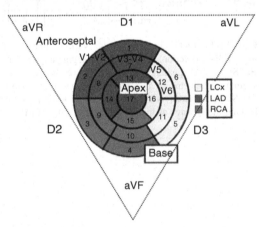

Fig. 11.16 Diagram showing the left ventricular segments, as defined by the American Heart Association, and their dependence on the three main braches of the coronary circulation. *LCx*, left circumflex artery; *LAD*, left anterior descending artery; *RCA*, right coronary artery (Modified from Cerqueria et al.)

Fig. 11.15 Anatomy of the coronary circulation. The right coronary artery (RCA) sends branches to the right atrium, the anterior wall of the right ventricle, the inferior wall of the left ventricle, one third of the posterior septum, the sinoatrial node (in 55% of cases), and the AV node (90% of cases), as well as to the posterior fascicle of the left bundle branch and the proximal segment of the bundle of His. The left anterior descending artery (LAD) supplies the anterior and anterolateral walls of the left ventricle, the remaining two thirds of the interventricular septum, the apex, the mid-anterior segment of the right ventricle, the lower third of the posterior septum of the right ventricle, the left atrium, the right bundle branch, and the anterior fascicle of the left bundle branch. The left circumflex artery supplies the lateral and (in 10% of cases) inferior walls of the left ventricle, the septal-perforating branch of the left bundle branch, the sinoatrial node (in 45% of cases), the AV node (in 10%), and sometimes the posterior fascicle of the left bundle branch. (Modified from Green, 2005)

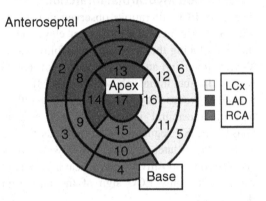

Fig. 11.17 Correlation between AHA-defined myocardial segments, ECG leads, and coronary vessels. *LCx*, left circumflex artery; *LAD*, left anterior descending artery; *RCA*, right coronary artery (Modified from Bayes de Luna et al.)

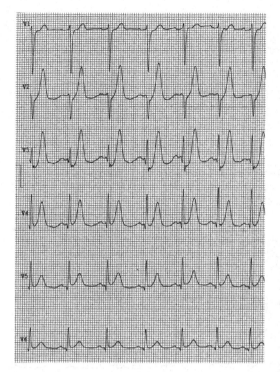

Fig. 11.18 Early stage of a anterior MI secondary to thrombotic occlusion of the proximal LAD: ST-segment depression, hyperacute T waves in the anterior leads, initial ST elevation in leads V5 and V6

In the earliest phases of a STEMI, the predominant ECG change will be hyperacute T waves (upright, high-voltage, and generally symmetrical) (Fig. 11.18). Only later will ST-segment elevation appear in the leads facing the ischemic area. It is important to note that in the initial phases, the most visible signs of damage may be *reciprocal changes*. Therefore, whenever ST depression is noted, one should always look carefully for even subtle ST elevation in the opposite leads. As noted above, its presence can have a major impact on management decisions.

Several points should be kept in mind when attempting to identify the "culprit" coronary artery on the basis of ECG findings. An inferior-wall infarction may be caused by occlusion of the right coronary artery (RCA) or the left circumflex artery (LCx), depending in which of the two is dominant. RCA involvement is suggested by ST elevation in lead III that is greater than that in lead II and associated with reciprocal ST depression in lead I. Vice versa, an LCx occlusion will produce greater ST elevation in lead II than in lead III with similar depression is leads V5, V6, and aVL and no reciprocal depression in lead I. In all AMIs—especially those involving the inferior wall—the right precordial leads (V3R, V4R) must be recorded to exclude involvement of the right ventricle. In some apical-anterior AMIs, Q waves may also be present in the inferior leads: in these cases, there is substantial inferior involvement because the left anterior descending artery (LAD), where the occlusion is located, is quite long, and the territory it supplies extends beyond the apex. In contrast, in septal AMIs, where inferior-wall involvement is generally more limited, RS or rS complexes will be recorded in leads II, III, and aVF.

Classification systems are naturally useful for obtaining a general picture of the damage, but there are frequent exceptions to the rules. Figures 11.19, 11.20, 11.21, 11.22, 11.23, 11.24, 11.25, 11.26, 11.27, 11.28, 11.29, 11.30, 11.31, 11.32, 11.33, 11.34, 11.35, 11.36, 11.37, 11.38, 11.39, 11.40, 11.41, 11.42, 11.43, and 11.44 show actual ECGs recorded during a variety of MIs (different stages, different areas of the infarction) with indications of the coronary vessels where the lesions were located.

Fig. 11.19 Acute
inferolateral MI with
ST-segment elevation in
the inferior leads (greater in
lead III than lead II) and
leads V3, V4, V5, and V6
and reciprocal ST
depression in lead aVL.
Cause: Nonocclusive
mid-segment thrombosis of
a large-caliber (approx.
5 mm) branch of the right
coronary artery and
thrombotic occlusion of the
LCx proximal segment

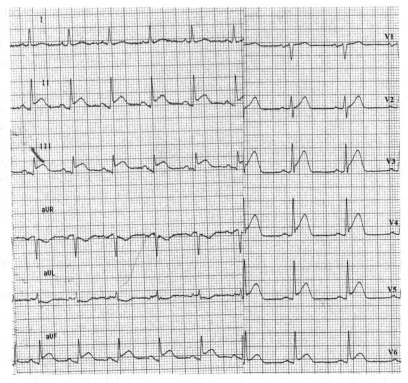

Fig. 11.20 Acute inferolateral MI secondary to occlusion of the proximal segment of right coronary artery. Q waves are already present in the inferior leads and in V5-V6, and lead V2 shows ST depression with high-voltage R waves. For years, infarctions of this type were classified as *posterior*, but in light of more recent findings, it is now classified as lateral-wall involvement (conclusion confirmed by echocardiography)

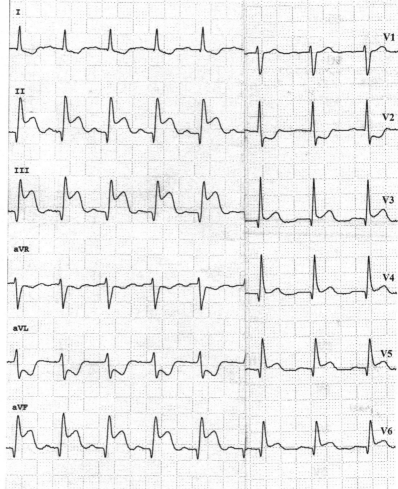

Fig. 11.21 Acute inferior MI with right ventricular involvement. (**a**) ST-segment elevation in the inferior leads. (**b**) Right precordial leads record QS complexes and ST elevation. The occlusion involved the middle segment of the right coronary artery

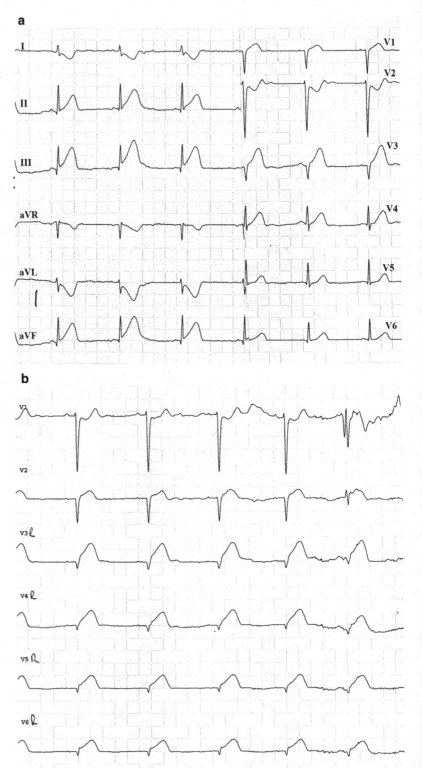

Fig. 11.22 Evolution of the case reported in Fig. 11.21. Q waves and negative T waves in inferior leads

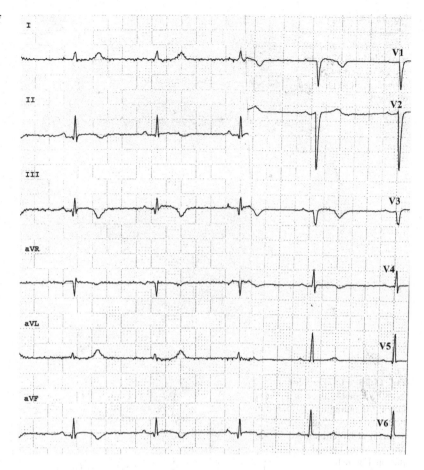

Fig. 11.23 Acute inferior MI caused by occlusion of a venous graft on the right coronary artery

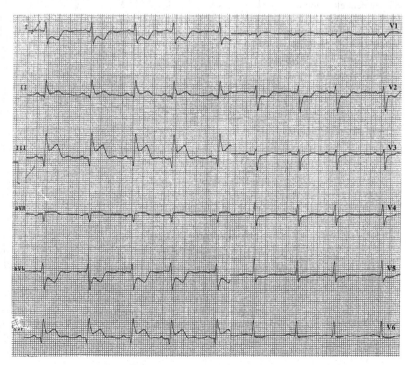

Fig. 11.24 Acute inferolateral MI (Q waves in the inferior leads, tall R waves in leads V2-V3) caused by mid-RCA occlusion. ECG recorded on day 3

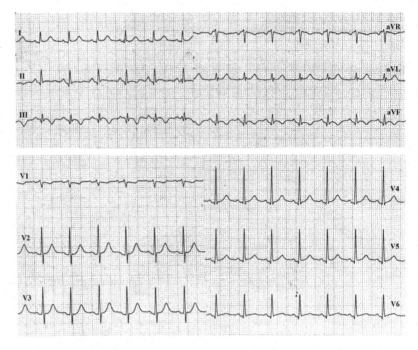

Fig. 11.25 ECG recorded in the hyperacute phase of a lateral MI caused by occlusion of the distal segment of left circumflex artery and the second diagonal branch. ST-segment elevation in leads I, aVL, V5, and V6 with ST depression in V1 through V4 and leads III and aVf. *Left*: Limb leads; *Right*: precordial leads

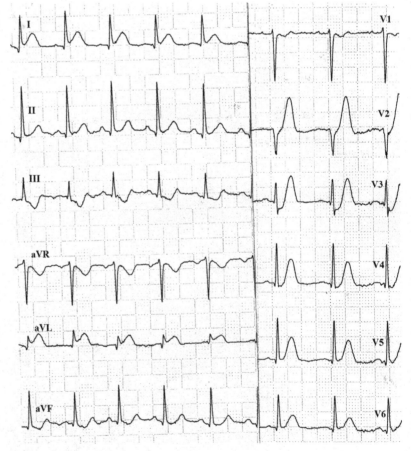

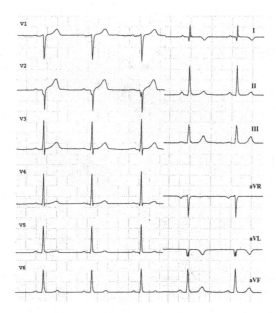

Fig. 11.26 Evolution of the MI shown in Fig. 11.25: QS complexes in V1, V2 and aVL; qR complexes in lead I. In the system proposed by Bayes de Luna, this is considered a mid-anterior MI because of the predominant involvement of the diagonal branch

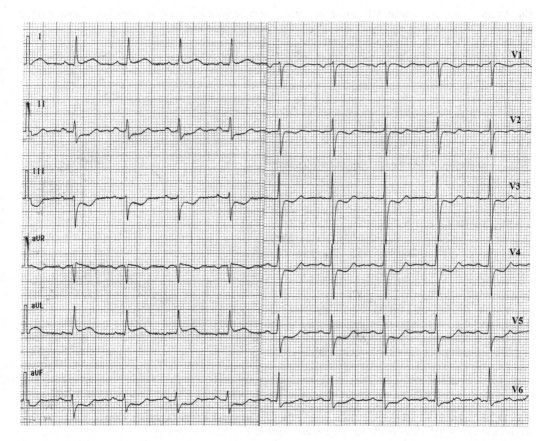

Fig. 11.27 Acute lateral MI caused by occlusion of the second diagonal branch. ST-segment elevation in leads I and aVL with reciprocal depression in the inferior and anterior leads

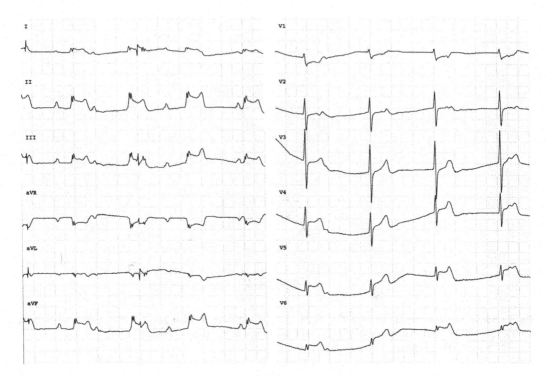

Fig. 11.28 Acute inferolateral MI caused by ostial occlusion of the circumflex artery and associated with complete AV block. The ST-segment elevation is seen in the inferior and lateral leads and is more pronounced in lead II than in lead III

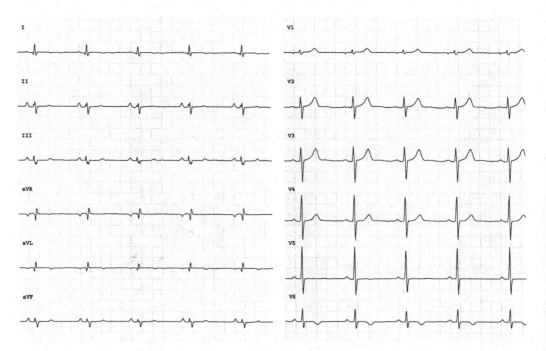

Fig. 11.29 Acute lateral MI secondary to a lesion of the large intermediate branch characterized by small q waves in leads I and aVL, tall R waves in V1, V2, and V3, and negative T waves in V5 and V6

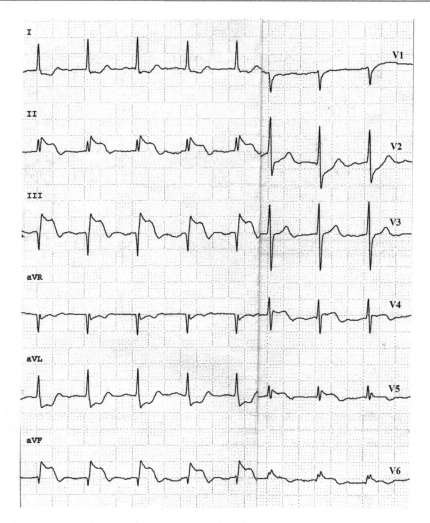

Fig. 11.30 Another acute inferolateral MI, this one caused by occlusion of the proximal segment of circumflex artery. ST-segment elevation in inferior leads and V4-V6. Tall R in V2 with depressed ST segment

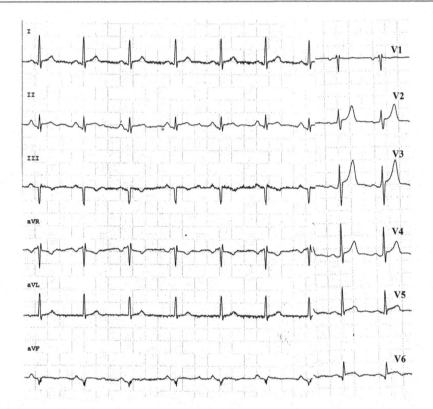

Fig. 11.31 Acute inferolateral MI. ECG obtained on day 4 shows reappearance of inferolateral ST-segment elevation (asymptomatic), possibly due to aneurysmal expansion of the lateral wall, which preceded electromechanical dissociation secondary to myocardial rupture on day 5

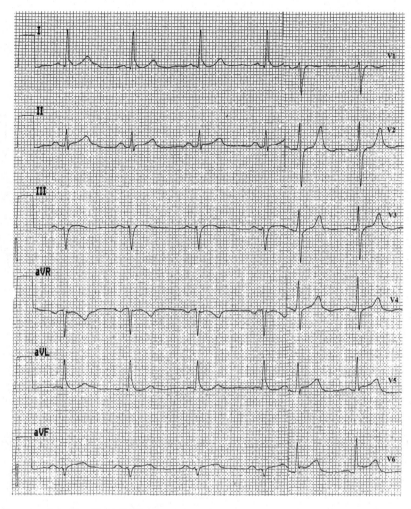

Fig. 11.32 Case shown in Fig. 11.31: ECG recorded at symptom onset shows ST elevation in V5-V6 and aVF with reciprocal ST depression in aVR

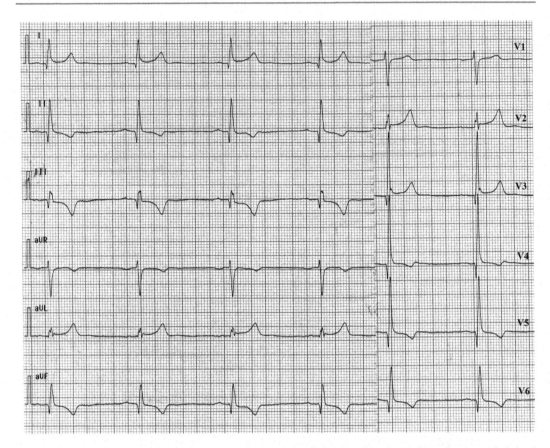

Fig. 11.33 Evolving inferolateral AMI caused by critical lesion of the distal segment of circumflex artery. Inferior Q waves in V5-V6, tall R waves in V2-V3

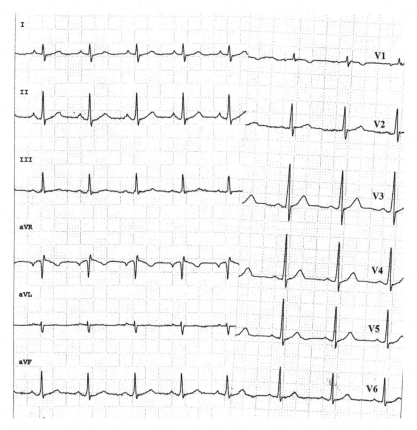

Fig. 11.34 Evolving lateral AMI caused by lesion of the proximal segment of circumflex artery. The only abnormal finding is a high-voltage R wave in leads V1-V3

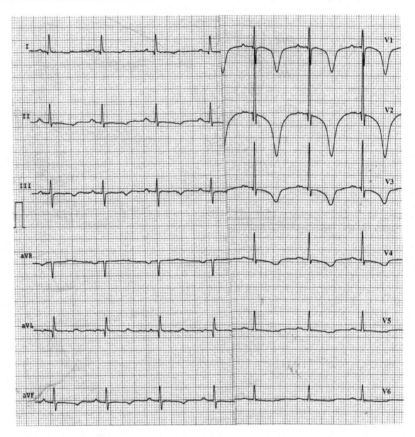

Fig. 11.35 Acute lateral MI caused by lesion of the first obtuse marginal branch. Tall R waves in V1-V3, anterior and inferior T-wave negativity with prolongation of the QT interval

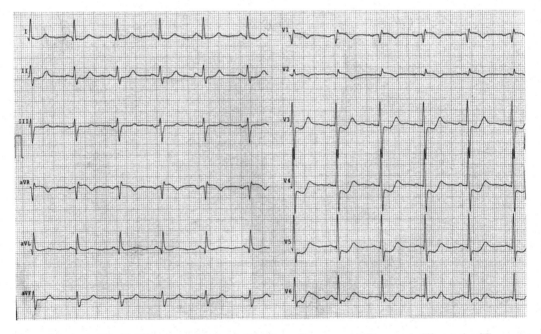

Fig. 11.36 Acute MI with ST-segment elevation in V1-V2, small q waves, tall R waves in V3, anterior ST segment depression. Critical lesion of the first diagonal branch, at its origin from the mid-LAD, associated with incomplete RBBB

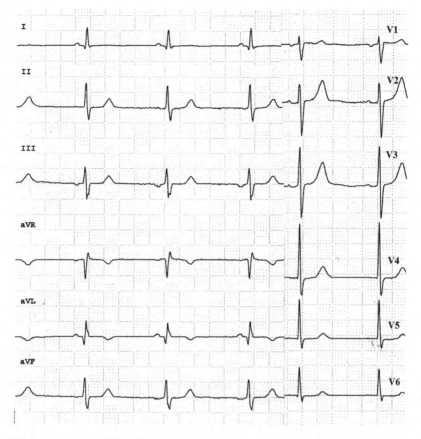

Fig. 11.37 Evolution of case shown in Fig. 11.36. Regression of incomplete RBBB: Tall R waves in V1-V3 and small Q waves in leads I and aVL. Findings indicative of a previous lateral MI

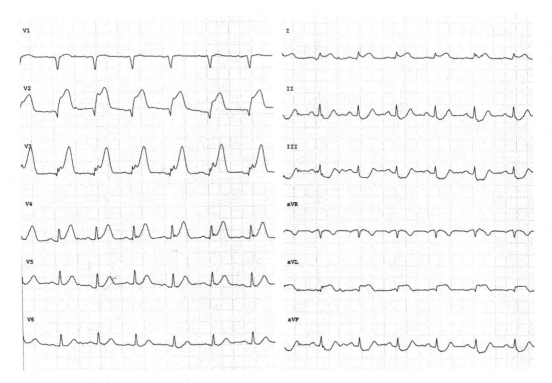

Fig. 11.38 Acute anterior MI secondary to occlusion of proximal segment of LAD. ST-segment elevation extends from V2 to leads V5, I, and aVL with reciprocal inferior depression

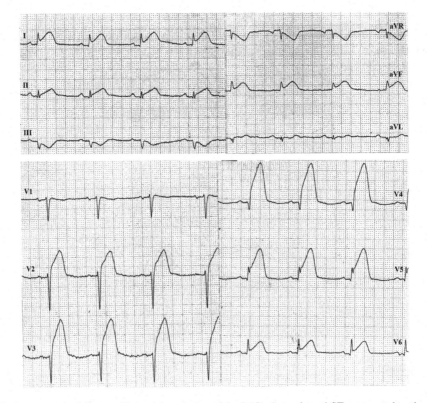

Fig. 11.39 Acute anterior MI caused by ostial occlusion of the LAD. Anterolateral ST-segment elevation

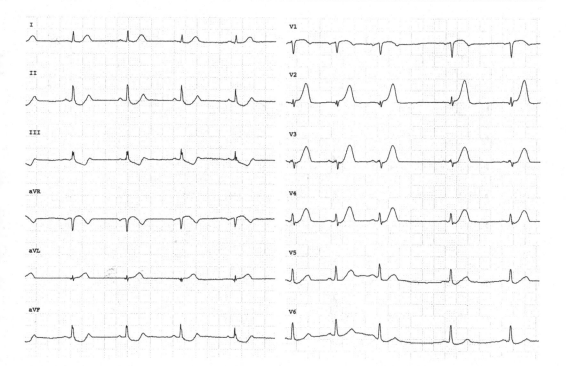

Fig. 11.40 Early ECG in another patient with acute anterior MI, this one caused by proximal occlusion of the LAD. Anterior hyperacute T waves with barely discernible ST elevation in leads V1-V2 and aVL. More informative is the obvious ST-segment depression in the inferior leads. It should prompt a careful search for signs of transmural ischemia, however subtle, since they will play a major role in treatment decisions

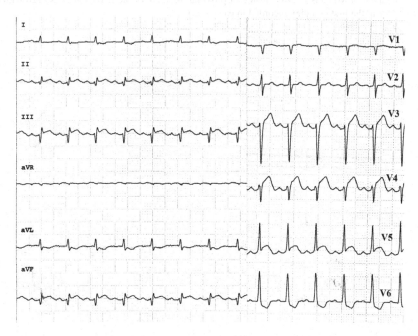

Fig. 11.41 Combined anterior-inferior MI caused by occlusion of the middle portion of the LAD, distal to the origin of the first diagonal branch. The right coronary artery is also occluded

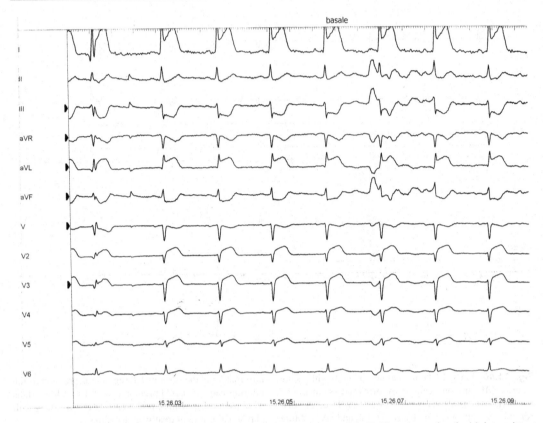

Fig. 11.42 Acute anterior MI caused by occlusion of proximal segment of the LAD and associated with intermittent RBBB (present only in the first complex recorded in each lead)

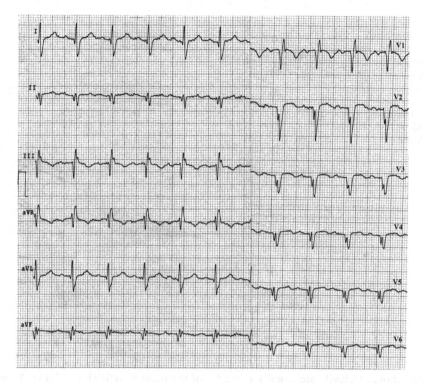

Fig. 11.43 Acute "U-shaped" (inferoanterior) MI extending far beyond the apex caused by occlusion of the middle portion of the LAD. Anterior QS and inferior Q waves. Complete RBBB and left anterior fascicular block (LAFB)

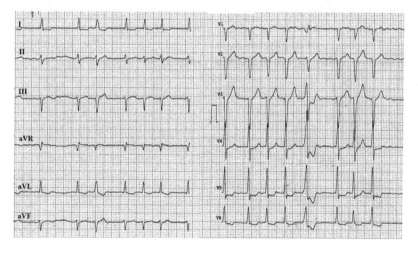

Fig. 11.44 Acute septal MI (QS in leads V1-V2) with atrial fibrillation. Nonocclusive lesion of the LAD at the level of the first septal branch

Fig. 11.45 Extensive
anterior AMI associated
with complete LBBB. The
ECG suggests proximal
segment thrombosis of the
LAD. Coronary
angiography revealed
patency of all the main
branches with no
significant lesions

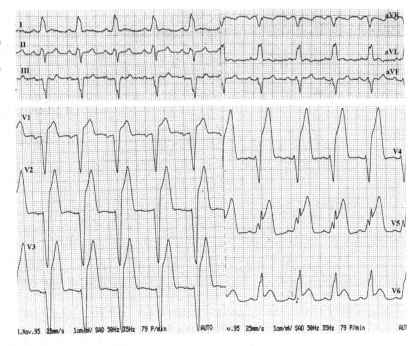

As noted above, STEMIs are usually caused by thrombotic occlusion of a coronary vessel. Much less commonly, the damage stems from protracted coronary artery spasm, sometimes associated with self-limited intracoronary thrombosis and no evidence of stenosis on cardiac catheterization. The coronary bed in these cases is lesion-free, but flow is often slowed in all three of the main vessels (Fig. 11.45). These findings probably reflect dysfunction of the coronary microcirculation that is severe enough to increase peripheral coronary resistance. This can also occur during coronary angioplasty as a result of peripheral microembolization by dislodged fragments of an atherothrombotic plaque (Fig. 11.46).

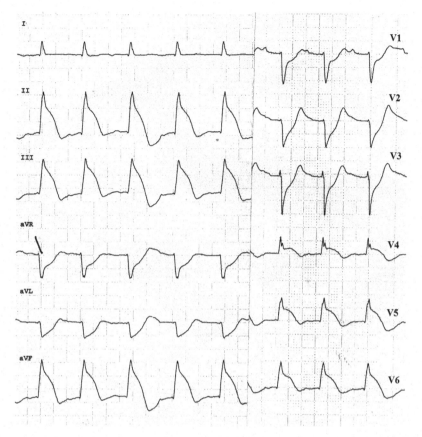

Fig. 11.46 Marked ST-segment elevation in inferior leads and V4-V6 in a patient who has just undergone coronary angioplasty for occlusion of the mid-proximal segment of circumflex artery. The ECG was recorded at the end of the procedure, when vessel patency and adequate flow had been restored. Transient electromechanical dissociation and complete AVB probably caused by severe left ventricular dysfunction secondary to peripheral microembolization. The ECG pattern remained unchanged for several hours despite restoration of effective systemic circulation

Complications of Infarction: ECG Findings

The complications of AMI reflected by changes in the ECG are numerous. Most involve arrhythmias, including all the types discussed in Chaps. 5 and 6. In the Figures that follow, tracings are shown that document complete AV blocks that developed *during* AMIs involving the inferolateral (Fig. 11.47), anterior (Fig. 11.48), and mid-anterior walls (Fig. 11.49). Figures 11.50 and 11.51 show atrial fibrillation and nodal supraventricular tachycardia, respectively, associated with inferior AMIs. The tracings shown in Figs. 11.52 and 11.53 were both recorded during anterior AMIs, the first complicated by ventricular tachycardia, the second by ventricular fibrillation.

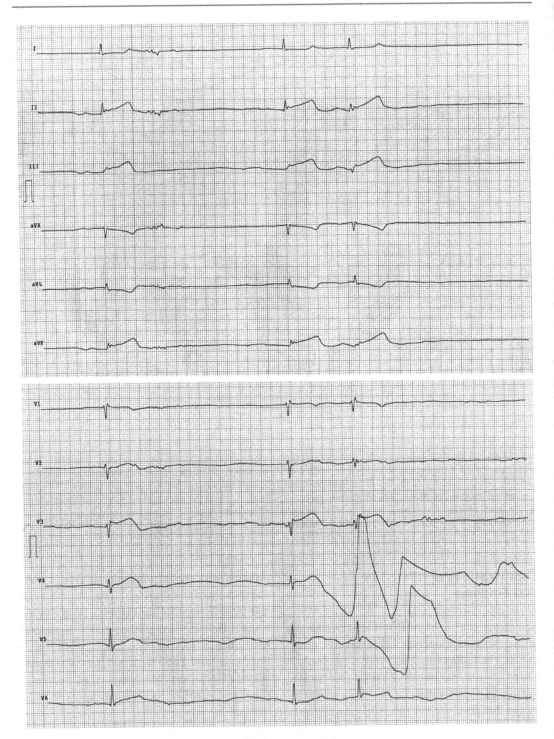

Fig. 11.47 Complete AVB in a patient with acute inferolateral MI secondary to ostial occlusion of the circumflex artery. Complete dissociation of atrial and ventricular activities and ST-segment elevation in inferior leads (II > III) and in V4-V6

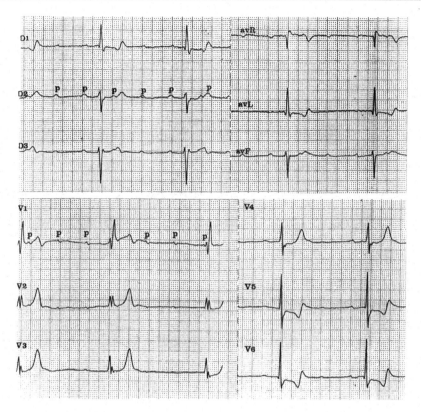

Fig. 11.48 Complete AVB during acute anterior MI. ST-segment elevation is present in V1 and hyperacute T waves in V2-V3

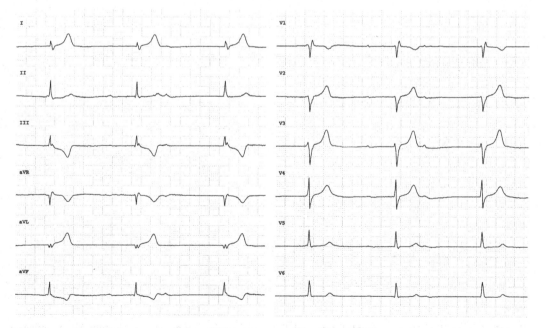

Fig. 11.49 Complete AVB during acute mid-anterior MI caused by occlusion of a large first diagonal branch arising from the LAD. Hyperacute T waves in leads V2-V3, I, and aVL. Q waves in aVL and V2 with minimal increase of the R wave amplitude in V3

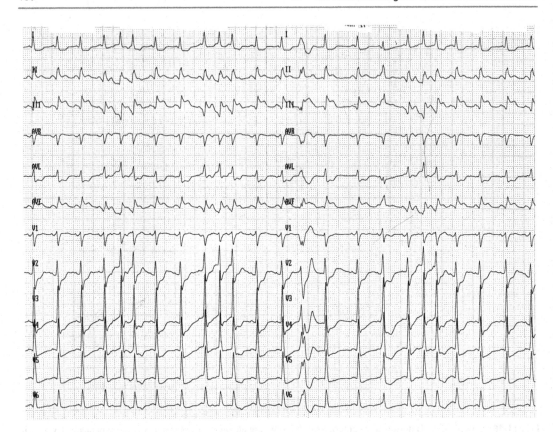

Fig. 11.50 Atrial fibrillation during acute inferior MI: ST-segment elevation in inferior leads, depression in anterior leads. Small q waves in inferior leads, tall R waves in V2

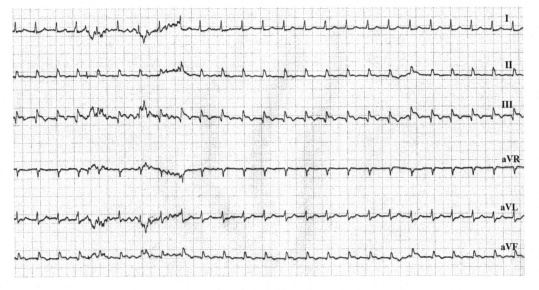

Fig. 11.51 Limb lead tracings recorded during SVT, probably nodal, during an acute inferior MI (ST-segment elevation in the inferior leads, reciprocal changes in leads I and aVL)

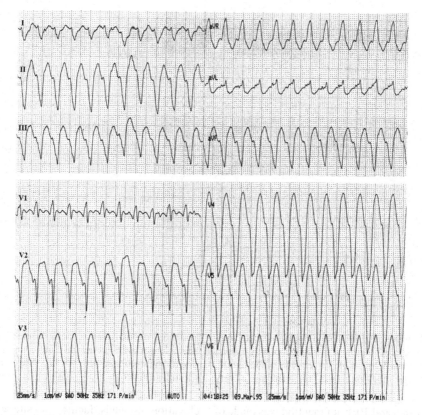

Fig. 11.52 Sustained ventricular tachycardia (see Chap. 6 for diagnostic criteria) during an acute anterior MI manifested by ST-segment elevation in precordial leads (V2 to V6) and inferior leads (lesion of the proximal LAD, whose distribution territory extends beyond the apex)

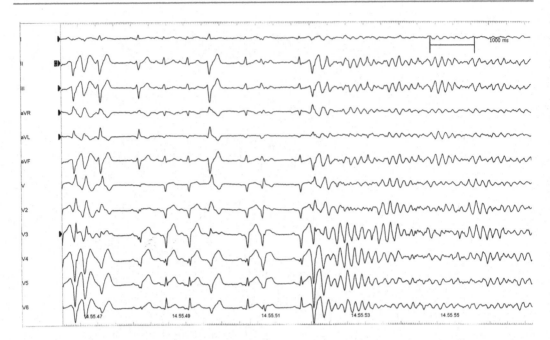

Fig. 11.53 Ventricular fibrillation during an acute anterior MI (ST-segment elevation in all precordial leads and Q waves in leads V1 through V4 left side of the figure). The ventricular fibrillation was triggered by a very premature ventricular extrasystole (R on T phenomenon) after a longer cycle (postextrasystolic pause). See discussion of afterdepolarizations in Chap. 6 for further electrophysiological details

In Chaps. 8 and 10, brief mention was made of the basic criteria used to diagnose AMIs associated with conduction disturbances and those occurring in patients with pacemakers. Examples of these situations are shown in Figs. 11.54, 11.55, and 11.56.

Mechanical complications can also cause specific ECG changes. Aneurysmal expansion of the left ventricle (especially the anterior wall and apex) is manifested by persistent ST-segment elevation in leads facing the site of necrosis (Fig. 11.57).

Distinctive ECG changes are also seen during phases characterized by severe left ventricular dysfunction (during cardiogenic shock, for example): they include QRS complexes with aberrant morphologies and repolarization changes, as in the case reported in Fig. 11.58, or during electromechanical dissociation (also referred to as pulseless electrical activity) (Figs. 11.59, 11.60, and 11.61).

Fig. 11.54 Acute anterior MI (ST-segment elevation of approx. 20 mm in V1, V2, V3, and V4) with complete LBBB

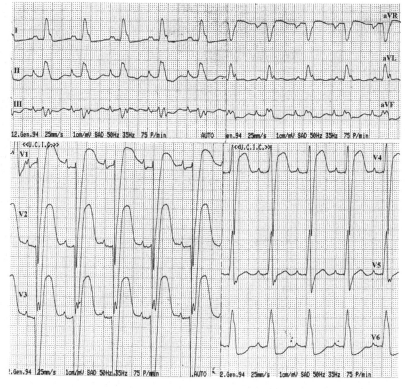

Fig. 11.55 Early phase of an acute anterior MI (anterior hyperacute T-wave with mild ST-segment elevation in leads V2 and V3) associated with complete RBBB

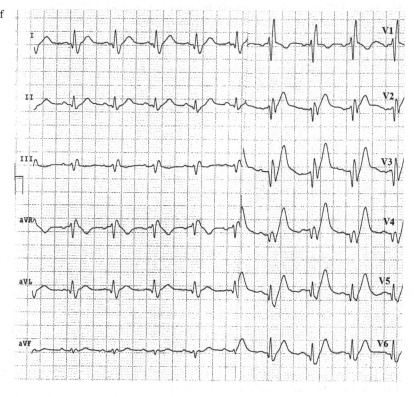

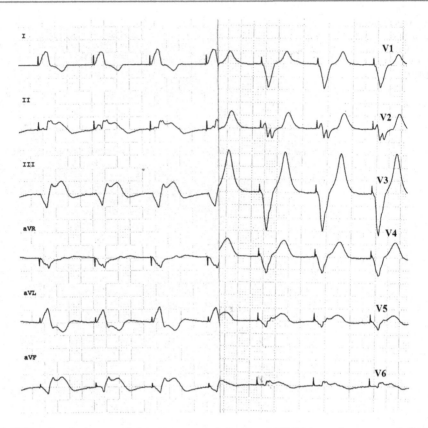

Fig. 11.56 VVI pacing rhythm recorded during an acute inferolateral MI. Pacing spikes are seen before each QRS complex and inferior ST-segment elevation is present in leads V5 and V6

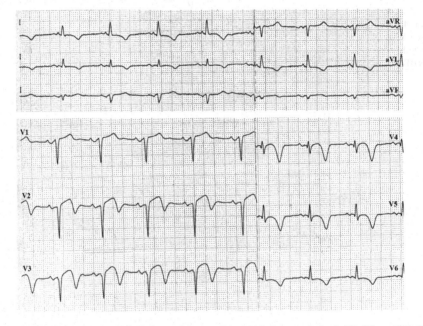

Fig. 11.57 Postinfarction aneurysm of the left ventricle associated with Q waves in leads V2, V3, and V4, ST-segment elevation, and diffuse anterolateral T-wave inversion

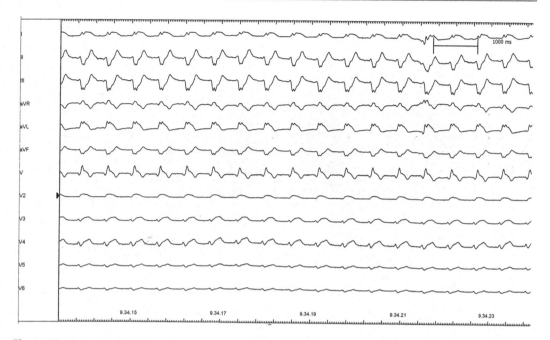

Fig. 11.58 Acute anterior MI caused by proximal occlusion of the LAD. Recanalization of the culprit artery was followed by no reflow, persistent left ventricular dysfunction, and the low cardiac output syndrome. The QRS complex displays marked aberrancy with complete RBBB and LAFB. Marked ST-segment elevation is seen in the anterior leads, especially leads I and aVL

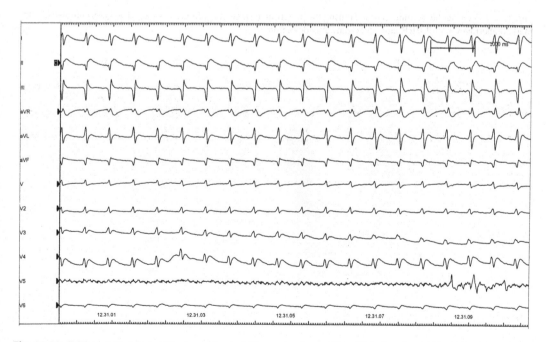

Fig. 11.59 ECG recorded during electromechanical dissociation caused by postinfarction cardiac rupture. The ventricular rhythm is completely dissociated from the nondiscernible atrial electric activity. Note the marked aberrancy of the QRS complex

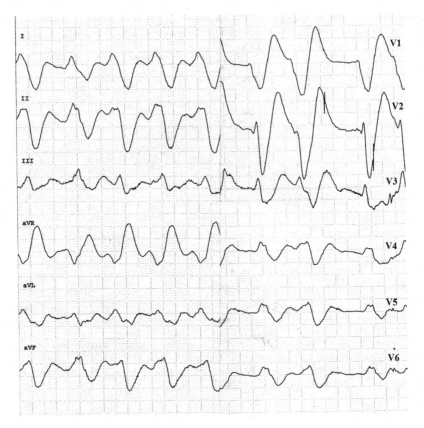

Fig. 11.60 Ventricular rhythm recorded during the preterminal stage of cardiogenic shock. The QRS complex displays marked aberrancy with LBBB and severe left axis deviation

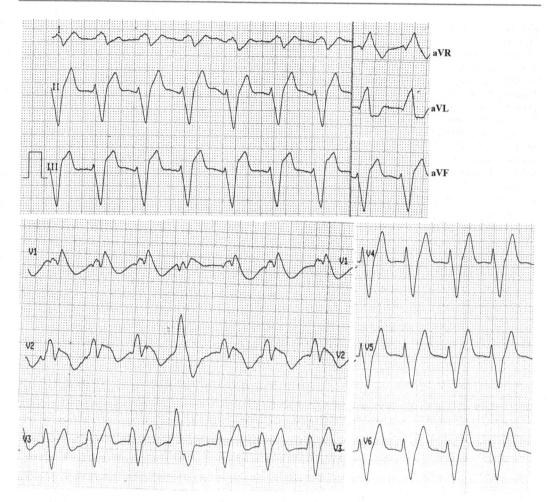

Fig. 11.61 Case similar to that shown in Fig. 11.60. Ventricular rhythm characterized by widened QRS with RBBB and LAFB patterns and ST-segment elevation in the inferoseptal leads. Acute anteroinferior MI

The Electrocardiogram During Coronary Angioplasty Procedures

The increasing use of percutaneous transluminal coronary angioplasty (PTCA) during acute coronary syndromes has improved our ability to correlate electrocardiographic changes with the specific coronary artery lesions causing the ischemia or infarct. It has also documented the ECG changes associated with the different phases of reperfusion, acute reocclusion, the no-reflow phenomenon (coronary patency after stenting but with markedly slowed or absent flow resulting in coronary thrombosis and severe ventricular dysfunction), and distal embolization of atherosclerotic plaque debris. The administration of contrast medium or intracoronary nitrates can also cause obvious albeit transient changes in the ECG.

Peripheral microembolism is probably the cause of the ECG changes shown in Fig. 11.62. The patient had an anteroseptal AMI treated with PTCA of the left anterior descending artery. The figure includes pre-procedure tracings and those recorded immediately after placement of a coronary stent, which was associated with transient ECG changes. Similar changes are seen in Figs. 11.63 and 11.64 (both recorded after PTCA on the LCx artery). This can also occur during elective PTCA, as shown in Fig. 11.65.

Fig. 11.62 Baseline ECG
(**a**) septal T wave inversion
with mildly increased
R-wave amplitude
reflecting necrosis.
Immediately after stent
placement (**b**), the T wave
changes become more
obvious, with prolongation
of the QT interval, and
more extensive, involving
leads V4, I, and aVL. Two
minutes later (**c**) the
baseline pattern is almost
fully restored

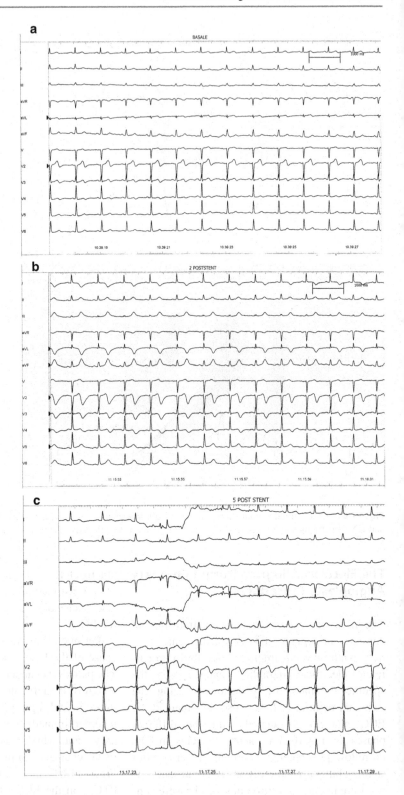

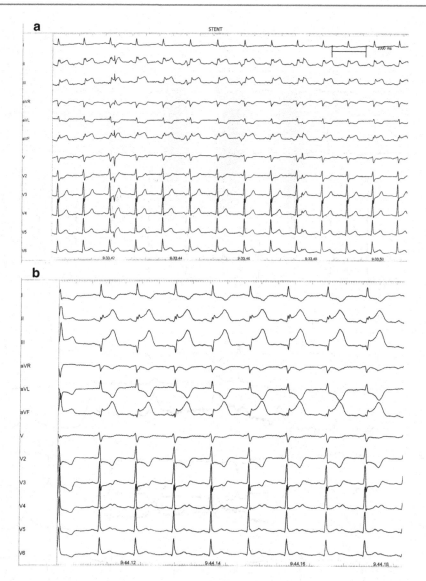

Fig. 11.63 Acute inferolateral MI (**a**) caused by occlusion of the mid-proximal segment of the circumflex artery (ST-segment elevation in the inferior leads and in leads V5 and V6 with ST-segment depression and tall R waves in V2). Restoration of vessel patency is immediately followed by (**b**) transient accentuation of the inferior ST-segment elevation, prolongation of the QT interval, and an increase in the amplitude of the QRS complex. Note reciprocal changes in leads I and aVL

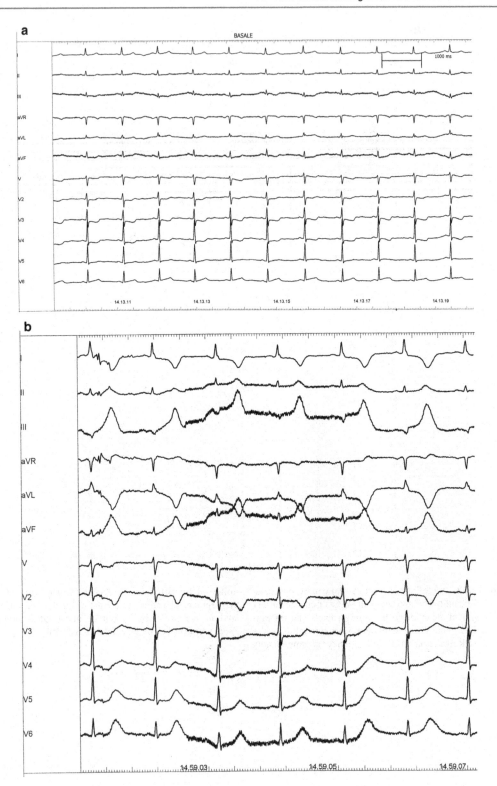

Fig. 11.64 Case similar to that shown in Fig. 11.63. ECG following PTCA of the mid-proximal segment of the circumflex artery. (a) ST-segment depression is seen in V1, V2, V3, and V4 and to a lesser extent in the inferior

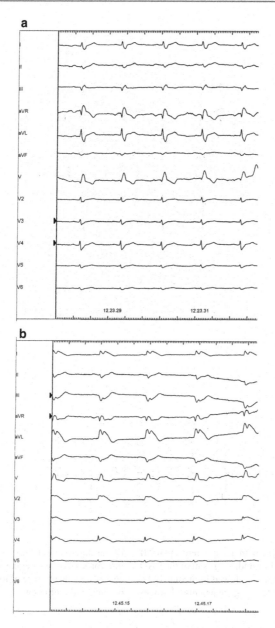

Fig. 11.65 Patient with exertional angina who underwent PCTA on the middle segment of LAD artery. The baseline ECG (**a**) shows RBBB and LAFB with an isoelectric ST segment. Stent implantation with probable peripheral embolization of plaque fragments was followed by (**b**) a transient anterolateral current of injury that distorts the QRS complex. Again, the changes were transient although they were associated with severe arterial hypotension

---

Fig. 11.64 (Continued) leads. This is a classic case in which one is likely to miss the subtle ST-segment elevation in leads V6 and aVL caused by complete occlusion of the LCx artery. The clue to its presence is the reciprocal ST-segment depression. (**b**) Stenting of the LCx artery is followed by marked prolongation of the QT interval and the appearance of hyperacute inferolateral T waves and T wave inversion in leads I and aVL. A few minutes later all alterations have disappeared

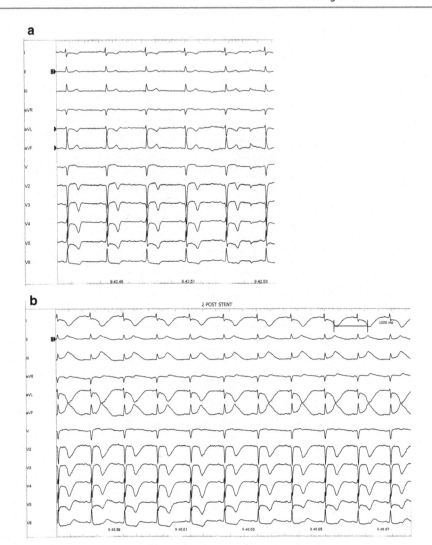

Fig. 11.66 ECG in a patient with acute anteroseptal MI caused by subocclusion of the middle segment of the LAD artery (**a**). Stent placement was followed immediately by (**b**) lengthening of the QT interval, giant negative T waves in the anterolateral regions, hyperacute T waves in the inferior regions. ST-segment elevation is seen in leads III and aVF in the absence of RCA involvement—suggestive of "inverted reciprocity"

Figure 11.66a shows a tracing from a patient with an acute anteroseptal MI caused by occlusion of the LAD. As shown in panel b of the same figure, PTCA was followed by the appearance of changes, which could have been interpreted, using the classic criteria, as inferior transmural ischemia with anterior reciprocity. The actual mechanism is the exact opposite. It is almost as if the reciprocity were inverted owing to the transient lengthening of the QT interval, which produces artifactual ST segment elevation in the inferior leads.

ECG changes can also appear when stent placement is followed by balloon dilation to optimize its expansion (Fig. 11.67).

Mention was made earlier of the no-reflow phenomenon after recanalization of an occluded coronary vessel: Fig. 11.68 shows a case in which reopening of the LAD was followed by severely reduced flow rates, which improved slowly after additional angioplasty.

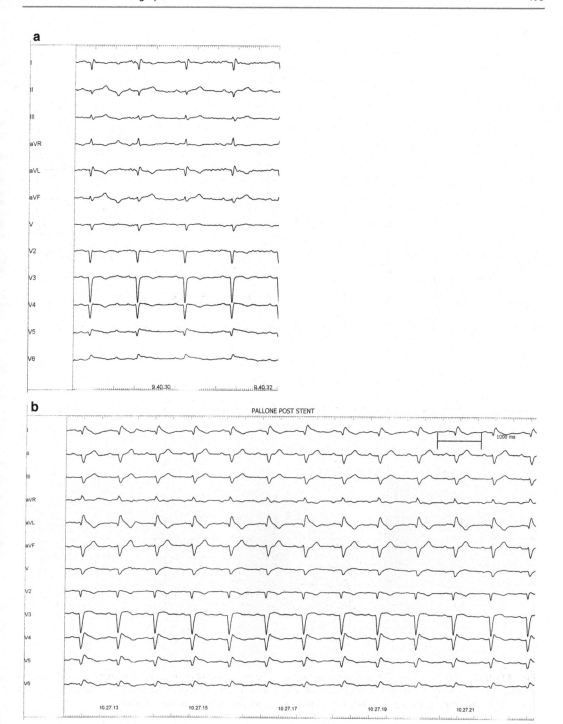

Fig. 11.67 The baseline ECG (**a**) shows signs of prior anterolateral-wall necrosis. Postdilatation of a stent implanted in the suboccluded venous graft on the oblique marginal artery was followed by (**b**) ST-segment elevation in the lateral leads associated with widening of the QRS complex indicative of a conduction disturbance. The changes are probably the result of transient ischemia caused by prolonged inflation of the balloon

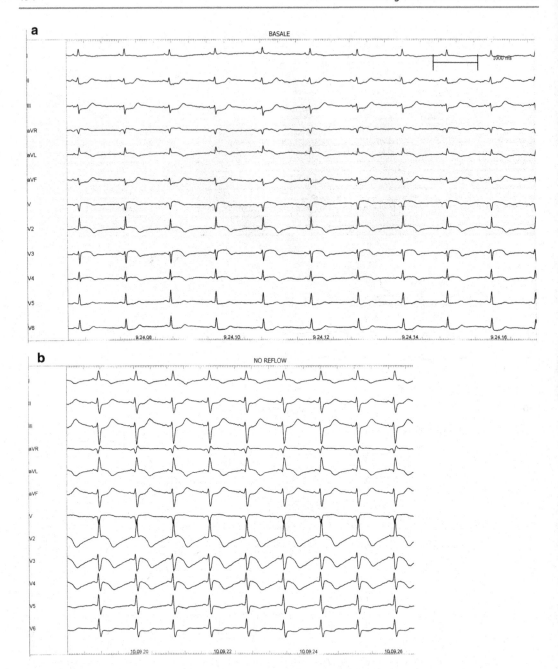

Fig. 11.68 Pre-PTCA tracing (**a**) indicative of acute anterior MI secondary to proximal occlusion of the LAD. The post-stenting tracing (**b**) shows evidence of the no-reflow phenomenon, with increased QRS amplitude, LAFB, and gross alterations of the ST-T segment with prolongation of the QT interval

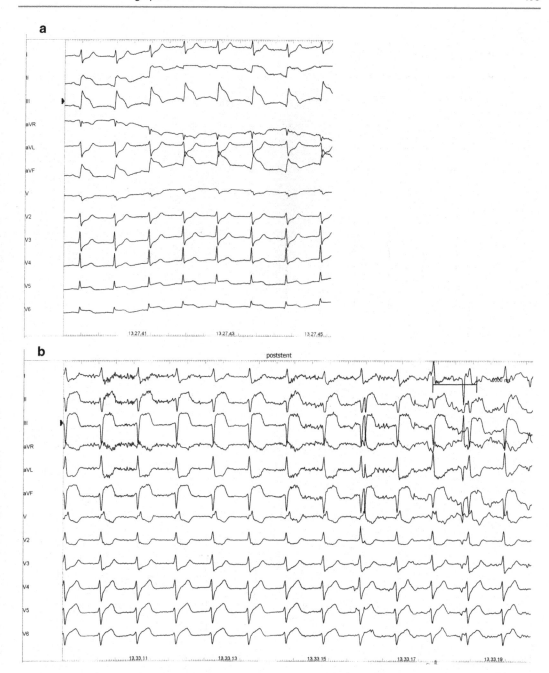

Fig. 11.69 ECGs recorded in a patient with an acute inferior MI caused by occlusion of the mid-distal segment of the right coronary artery. The initial tracing (**a**) shows inferolateral ST-segment elevation and a vertical electrical axis. After PTCA (**b**) evidence of RBBB and LAFB appeared with persistent inferolateral ST-segment elevation and anterior ST-segment depression

Transient conduction disturbances can also be seen after PTCA. They are probably caused by peripheral embolization phenomena (Fig. 11.69).

The administration of intracoronary nitrates may also be followed by gross, transient changes in the ECG, which may be related to

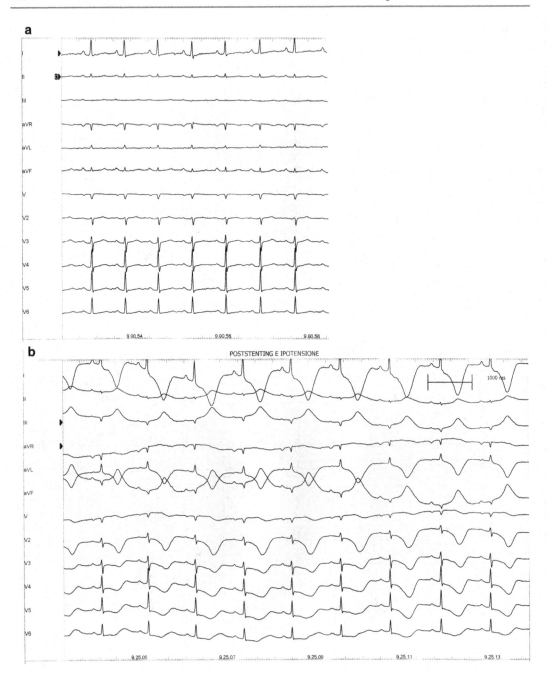

Fig. 11.70 ECGs recorded in a patient with unstable angina caused by a critical lesion of the middle circumflex artery. The baseline tracing (**a**) shows no significant changes. Implantation of a stent and intracoronary nitrate infusion (**b**) was followed by gross changes in repolarization (giant negative T waves in the anterolateral region, hyperacute T waves in the inferior region), marked lengthening of the QT interval, and an increase in the amplitude of the QRS complex. The patient also had severe arterial hypotension

maldistribution of the blood flow (steal mechanism), as shown in Fig. 11.70. In the post-infusion tracing, it is also important to note the markedly prolonged QT interval, which some authors consider an early sign of transmural ischemia. A similar phenomenon is seen in the post-stenting tracing shown in Fig. 11.68.

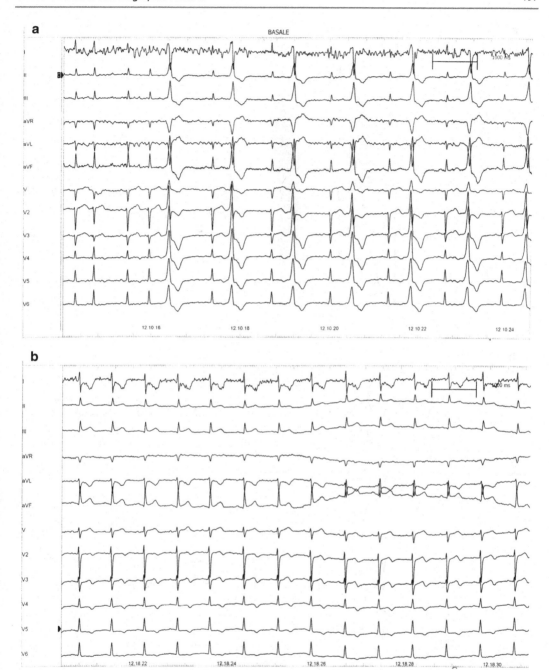

Fig. 11.71 ECG recorded in a patient with acute coronary syndrome caused by critical lesion of the LAD. The baseline ECG (**a**) shows minor alterations of repolarization, frequent ventricular extrasystoles, and a vertical electrical axis. Injection of contrast medium into the patent right coronary artery (**b**) induces ST-segment elevation in the inferior leads, reciprocal ST-segment depression in leads I and aVL, and anterior T-wave inversion. Note also the appearance of R waves in V1-V3, which may reflect mild disturbance of conduction along the right bundle branch

Intracoronary injection of contrast medium can also cause ECG changes, even in the absence of coronary lesions (Fig. 11.71). The mechanism underlying these changes in not completely clear: it seems to be related to the contrast medium's ability to prolong the action potential and cause dispersion of ventricular repolarization. This might explain the findings shown in Fig. 11.72.

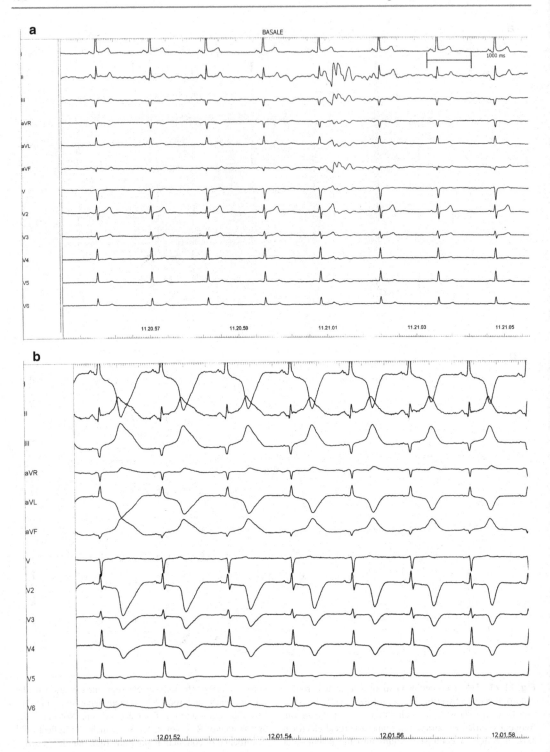

Fig. 11.72 ECG recorded in a patient with unstable angina secondary to critical lesion of the proximal segment of LAD. (**a**) Barely discernible ST-segment elevation in leads I and aVL with reciprocal depression in leads III and aVF. (**b**) Injection of contrast medium into the LAD causes a substantial increase in the amplitude of the QRS, prolongation of the QT interval, inferior T-wave positivization and anterolateral negativization

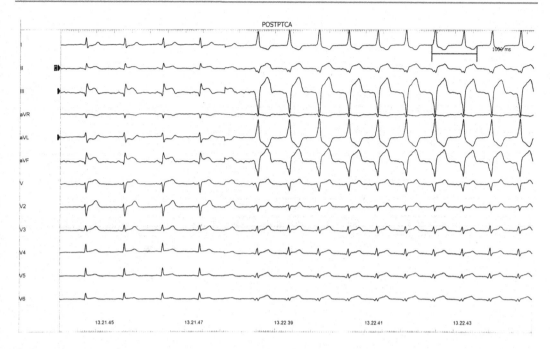

Fig. 11.73 ECG recorded during PCTA in a patient with acute inferior MI caused by proximal RCA occlusion. Advancing the guide wire into the occlusion allows reperfusion of the infarcted area, which is heralded by the onset of an accelerated idioventricular rhythm

And finally, a phenomenon that is not a complication but a prognostically positive sign: the onset of an accelerated idioventricular rhythm. This reperfusion arrhythmia is triggered by the simple passage of the guide wire through the lumen of the occluded coronary vessel, a maneuver capable of producing partial reperfusion of the infarcted territory (Fig. 11.73).

Cardiac Chamber Hypertrophy

12

Atrial Abnormalities

General Considerations

In the past, P-wave anomalies associated with cardiac chamber hypertrophy have been referred to with a variety of terms, which reflected their origins in specific anatomic or physiological alterations of one or both atria. In reality, however, the diverse underlying mechanisms often produced similar, virtually indistinguishable changes at the level of the ECG, and for this reason, the less specific term *atrial abnormality*, rather than atrial hypertrophy or enlargement, was recommended in 2009 by the American Heart Association Electrocardiography and Arrhythmias Committee, Council on Clinical Cardiology; the American College of Cardiology Foundation; and the Heart Rhythm Society, and it will be used in this chapter.

Atrial abnormalities reflect pressure or volume overload of the atria—the former secondary to obstructed outflow (e.g., mitral valve stenosis), the latter to atrioventricular valve insufficiency or shunting. Regardless of its original cause, the overload tends to develop mixed features over time. The electrocardiographic changes become obvious in the more advanced stages, particularly when there is a combined pressure and volume overload, which causes substantial atrial dilatation capable of augmenting the electric potentials.

Right Atrial Abnormality

Right atrial abnormality is generally manifested by increases in both the amplitude and duration of the right atrial action potentials. The recorded P wave represents the sum of the right atrial component with that of the left atrium (Fig. 12.1), which begins and ends after the former. For this reason, in the presence of an enlarged right atrium, the amplitude of the P wave is increased but its duration is not appreciably prolonged.

The P waves in leads II, III, and aVF become tall and pointed, with an amplitude of >2.5 mm (Fig. 12.2). In leads V1 and V2, the P wave may be unchanged or it may become pointed (positive or biphasic with predominance of the initial positivity). The right atrial abnormality is sometimes so pronounced that it displaces the right ventricle, which is also dilated in many cases. The QRS morphology varies (QR, Qr, or qR complexes with no evidence of LBBB or prior necrosis).

Left Atrial Abnormality

The opposite pattern occurs when the left atrium is involved. The potentials that are amplified (in terms of amplitude and duration) are those related to the second component of atrial activation. As a result, the overall duration of the P wave is increased (110 ms in adults, >90 ms in children), and its morphology reflects

Fig. 12.1 Right atrial abnormality—Increased amplitude of the first component of the P wave in the frontal and horizontal planes. In the frontal plane, the amplitude of the second vector diminishes and that of the first vector increases. Compare P-wave components in a healthy subject shown in Fig. 3.2

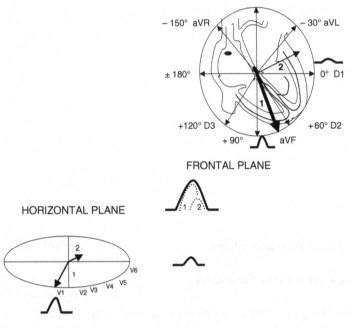

FRONTAL PLANE

HORIZONTAL PLANE

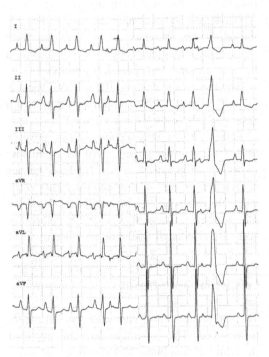

Fig. 12.2 Patient with primary pulmonary hypertension and right ventricular hypertrophy. The ECG shows a P wave with normal duration (<100 ms) and an amplitude of approximately 4 mm and a biphasic configuration in lead V1 with predominance of the first component

predominance of the terminal forces of atrial activation, particularly in lead V1.

The main P-wave abnormalities are left axis deviation (P-wave axis 0° to +30°), duration of more than 110 ms, a biphasic waveform in V1-V2 with predominance of the terminal negativity, a notched waveform in leads I, II, and aVL with an amplitude increase in the second component (the so-called *P-mitrale*) (Fig. 12.3). In addition to their increased duration, the P waves recorded in leads II, aVF, V3, and V4 are widely notched with peaks separated by 40 ms or more (Fig. 12.4).

Combined Right- and Left-Atrial Abnormality

In this case, the ECG changes will be a combination of the alterations discussed above. In leads I, II, and aVL, the P waves will be widely notched (as they are in left atrial abnormality), and the initial component will be tall and pointed (reflecting right atrial abnormality). Lead V1 may record a biphasic P wave with accentuation of the positive initial component (right atrial abnormality) and of the negative terminal component (caused by left atrial abnormality).

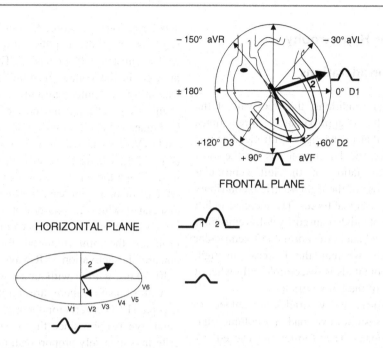

Fig. 12.3 Left atrial abnormality—Alteration of the second component of the P wave, which is predominant in both the frontal and horizontal planes

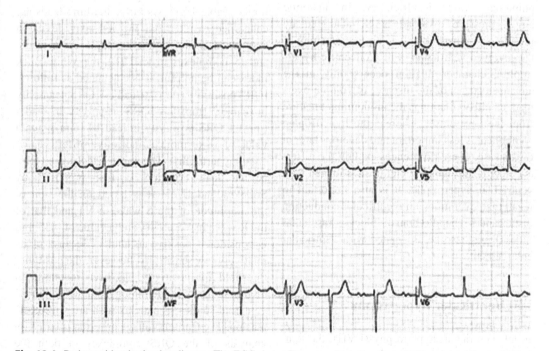

Fig. 12.4 Patient with mitral valve disease: The ECG shows P waves with a duration of 120 ms, notching in the limb leads, and predominance of the negative component in V1

Ventricular Hypertrophy

General Considerations

Under normal conditions, the free wall of the Left ventricle is approximately three times thicker than that of the right ventricle. For this reason, the ventricular complex is for the most part a representation of the left ventricular potentials; those of the right ventricle contribute mainly to the terminal forces. The increase in left ventricular potentials caused by left ventricular hypertrophy enhances the normal left ventricular predominance, whereas the increase in right ventricular potentials is discernible only when it exceeds that of the left ventricle.

Like the atria, the ventricles are subject to pressure (or systolic) overload and volume (diastolic) overload. The former is caused by obstructed ejection (typically associated with aortic valve stenosis, systemic or pulmonary hypertension). Pressure overload is caused by aortic or pulmonary valve insufficiency. In anatomic terms, pressure overload is characterized by muscle-cell hypertrophy leading to thickening of the involved ventricular wall (concentric hypertrophy); chamber dilation occurs only in the advanced stages of the disease. In volume overload, chamber dilation is the predominant feature from the very outset, whereas the hypertrophic component is less important and develops later in the disease. These differences explain the different electrocardiographic pictures associated with ventricular hypertrophy. It is also important to recall that, over time, intraventricular conduction disturbances (bundle-branch blocks, fascicular blocks) may also be associated with ventricular enlargement.

Left Ventricular Hypertrophy

In left ventricular hypertrophy (LVH), the temporal sequence of the three phases of ventricular depolarization is normal, but the voltage resulting from the depolarization of the free wall is substantially increased. There is also in increase in the voltage resulting from depolarization of the interventricular septum. These changes are reflected on the electrocardiogram by higher-voltage R waves in the left precordial leads (V5-V6) and deeper S waves in V1-V2 (Fig. 12.5). Changes are also seen in the limb leads facing the left ventricle (leads I and aVL), which display increased-voltage R waves associated with left axis deviation (to $-20°$ or $-30°$). The increased myocardial mass also prolongs the time required for endocardial-epicardial activation (R-wave peak time >40–50 ms, with or without a q wave).

Unfortunately, there are no internationally accepted ECG criteria for diagnosis of left ventricular hypertrophy since the sensitivity of most criteria is inversely proportional to their rigidity. Those related to QRS voltage are the ones most widely used, but they apply mainly to adults whose heights and weights are within normal limits (Table 12.1). As far as the limb leads are concerned (aside from the left axis deviation mentioned above with qR complexes in lead I and rS complexes in lead III), the White-Bock index can be helpful. It is calculated as follows: [QRS positivity (mm) in lead I + QRS negativity in lead III (mm)] − [QRS negativity in lead I (mm) + QRS positivity in lead III (mm)], and a value of 18 or more is indicative of left ventricular hypertrophy. The most widely used precordial lead criterion is that proposed by Sokolow and Lyon. It is based on the sum of the amplitude of the S wave in V1 and that of the R wave in V5 or V6, and a value of ≥35 mm is considered positive in adults. Because of its relatively low sensitivity, however, the positivity threshold for positivity has been increased to 38 mm in recent epidemiologic studies and interventional studies of patients with arterial hypertension. The Cornell voltage criterion is based on analysis of the QRS complexes in both the precordial and limb leads. It is the sum of the

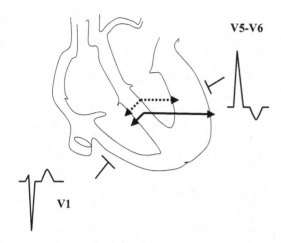

Fig. 12.5 In LVH, increase in the thickness of the left ventricle alters the ventricular activation vector (compare *bold arrows* with *dotted arrows* representing the normal vectors). As a result, large-amplitude R waves are seen the left precordial leads and deep S waves in V1

Table 12.1 Criteria for diagnosing left ventricular hypertrophy

– Sokolow-Lyon: $S_{V1} + R_{V5 \text{ or } V6} > 38$ mm

– Cornell Voltage: $R_{aVL} + S_{V3} > 20$ mm (F), >25 mm (M)

– Product of the Cornell Voltage × QRS duration > 2440 mm/ms

– White-Bock index: (R I + S III) − (S I + R III) > 18

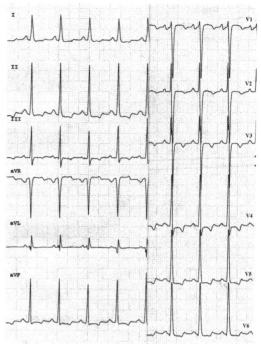

Fig. 12.6 This ECG meets all of the main criteria for diagnosis of LVH: increased R-wave voltage in the precordial leads (Sokolow-Lyon index 48 mm, Cornell voltage 30 mm, product QRS duration × Cornell voltage 3000 mm/ms), R-peak time 60 ms, left atrial abnormality. The repolarization phase shows the effects of the overload (asymmetric negative T waves in the left precordial leads with mild ST-segment depression)

amplitudes of the S wave in V3 and the R wave in aVL. Values above 20 mm (females) or 25 mm (males) are indicative of left ventricular hypertrophy. The low sensitivity of criteria based exclusively on voltage has prompted the development of others which also consider the duration of the QRS complex, which increases with the degree of hypertrophy. One example is the product of the QRS duration and the Cornell voltage (plus 6 mm for women). Values exceeding 2440 mm/ms are indicative of left ventricular hypertrophy.

With the progression of hypertrophy, alterations involving repolarization may also appear in the leads facing the left ventricle. They tend to develop earlier in the presence of systolic rather than diastolic overload. This ECG picture, referred to as strain, is characterized by the presence in leads V5 and V6 of asymmetrical T-wave inversions, sometimes associated with upwardly convex ST-segment depression. Left atrial abnormality may also be present (Fig. 12.6).

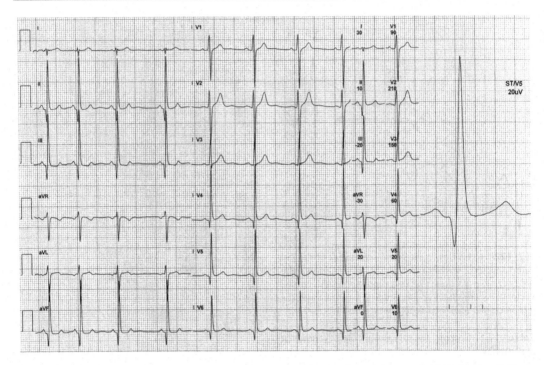

Fig. 12.7 LVH secondary to moderate aortic valve insufficiency. The ECG meets the criteria of Schamroth regarding the increased amplitude of the QRS complex, the presence of septal Q waves in the left precordial leads and the mild upwardly concave ST-segment elevation in V6

In patients with diastolic overload, the long-term picture (described by Leo Schamroth in the 1970s) is characterized by an increased QRS amplitude, the presence of septal Q waves in the left precordial leads, and mild upwardly concave ST-segment elevation in V6 (Fig. 12.7). In some cases, advanced left ventricular hypertrophy is also associated with left bundle-branch conduction disturbances, such as complete LBBB (Fig. 12.8) or left anterior fascicular block (LAFB).

Right Ventricular Hypertrophy

Most conditions that give rise to right ventricular hypertrophy are capable of provoking systolic overload of this ventricle. The increased right ventricular mass is associated with an appreciable voltage increase during depolarization of the right ventricular free wall, which is reflected mainly by tall R waves in V1 and V2 (Fig. 12.9).

Axis deviation is evident in the limb leads: as the overload increases, the axis shifts progressively to the right, with rS complexes in lead I and qR complexes in lead III. As the hypertrophy progresses, lead aVR exhibits QR or qR complexes. These changes are accompanied by the appearance or accentuation of S waves in V6. Mild-to-moderate right ventricular hypertrophy is not associated with T-wave changes. In the advanced stages, however, T-wave inversion occurs in opposition to the R waves, first in V1-V3 and later also in leads III and aVF.

The most informative aspect of the ECG is the dominant R wave in V1 and V2, whose voltage

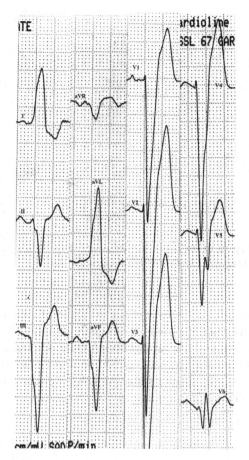

Fig. 12.8 LVH associated with complete LBBB in a patient with severe aortic stenosis. Even in the presence of the LBBB, the diagnosis of LVH can be made on the basis of the voltage features and left axis deviation

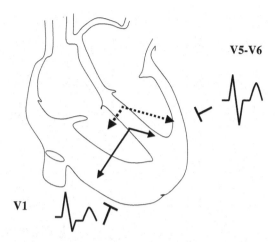

Fig. 12.9 In RVH, increase in the thickness of the right ventricular myocardium alters the ventricular activation vector (compare *bold arrows* with *dotted arrows* representing the normal vectors), increasing the amplitude of the R waves seen in V1 and V2 and that of the S wave in V5 and V6

increases as the systolic overload becomes more severe.

The QRS morphology most commonly seen in lead V1 is an Rs or RS complex, although small q waves reflecting extension of the hypertrophy into the upper portion of the interventricular septum are by no means rare (Fig. 12.10). The rsR' configuration can be seen in patients with moderate overload (Fig. 12.11).

In the present of severe right atrial hypertrophy, the right ventricle is often dilated (e.g., secondary to pulmonary embolism) and

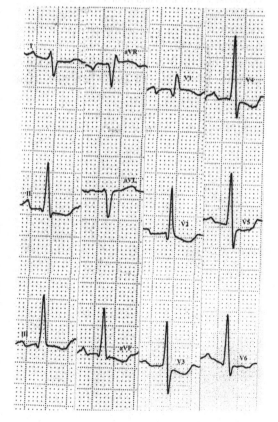

Fig. 12.10 ECG in a patient with mitral valve stenosis and secondary pulmonary hypertension. qR complexes are see in V1 and V2, along with ST-segment depression in the inferior leads and in V1 through V4, right axis deviation (axis +120°), left atrial abnormality (negativity of the second P wave component in V1)

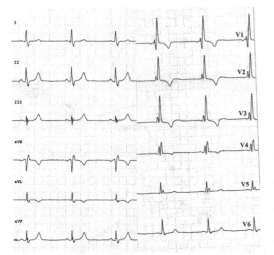

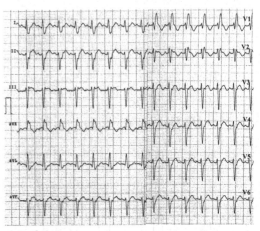

Fig. 12.12 ECG in an individual with a large atrial septal defect and complete RBBB with left axis deviation

Fig. 12.11 ECG in a patient with moderate pulmonary valve stenosis: typical findings include right bundle-branch block (RBBB) with an rsR′ morphology in V1-V3 and T-wave inversion from V1 through V4

sometimes rotated posteriorly. In these cases, there may be QR, Qr, or qR complexes, in the absence of LBBB or signs of prior myocardial necrosis (see Fig. 14.2). When the right ventricular hypertrophy is the result of volume overload, the most characteristic alteration is a variable delay in right ventricular activation, which displays poor correlation with the hemodynamic status of the pulmonary circulation (Fig. 12.12).

The Electrocardiogram in Diseases of the Pericardium and Myocardium

13

Acute Pericarditis

Acute pericarditis is associated with inflammation of the subepicardial layers of the myocardium, which are in contact with the pericardium. The electrocardiogram (ECG) can be useful in the diagnosis of this disorder, revealing diffuse ST-segment and T-wave changes that evolve in a characteristic manner and are phase-specific.

Within a few hours of symptom onset, ST-segment elevation appears. It reflects abnormal repolarization secondary to pericardial inflammation and is the most sensitive ECG criterion for pericarditis. The ST-segment elevation is diffuse and concordant with the T waves. Its magnitude (the amplitude rarely exceeds 5 mm) and upwardly concave shape distinguish it from the convex ST-segment elevation associated with transmural ischemia. The ST-segment alterations associated with acute pericarditis are generalized because the pericardial inflammation is usually diffuse. ST-segment elevation is never observed in lead aVR, but ST-segment depression may well be present in lead aVR or V1 (Fig. 13.1). Acute pericarditis can also be distinguished from acute myocardial infarction by the absence of reciprocal ST-segment depression in leads opposite to those displaying elevation and by the invariable absence of necrosis-related Q waves (excluding those reflecting a prior infarction). During this phase, the presence of a significant pericardial effusion leads to diffuse reductions in the amplitudes of all electrocardiographic waves owing to the electrical insulating effects of the large fluid collection (Fig. 13.2). In subsequent phases, the ST-segment elevation diminishes, and T-wave inversion appears. It can persist for long periods of time but disappears as the clinical picture improves (Fig. 13.3).

M. Romanò, *Text Atlas of Practical Electrocardiography*,
DOI 10.1007/978-88-470-5741-8_13, © Springer-Verlag Italia 2015

Fig. 13.1 Acute
pericarditis. Diffuse
ST-segment elevation with
ST-segment depression in
V1 and aVR

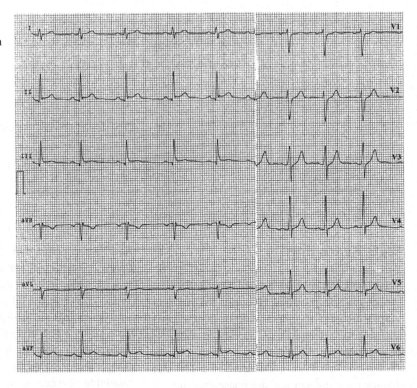

Fig. 13.2 ECG in a patient
with massive pericardial
effusion causing
pericardial tamponade. The
key feature is a significant
decrease in the QRS
voltage in all leads

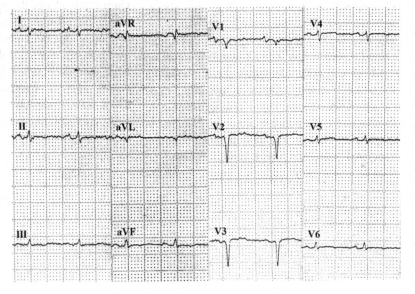

Fig. 13.3 Evolution of the ECG picture associated with acute pericarditis shown in Fig. 13.2. Inferolateral ST-segment elevation persists but is less marked, and negative T waves have appeared in the same leads

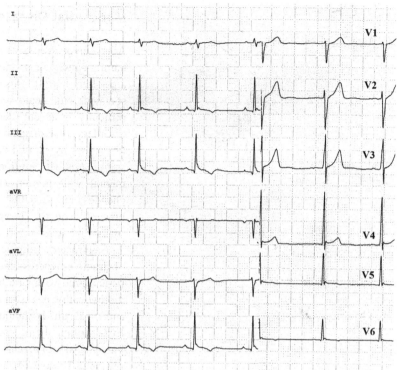

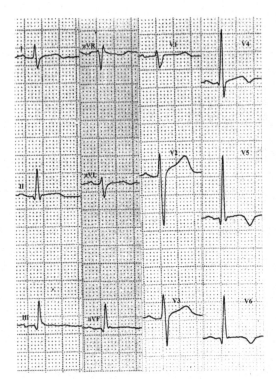

Fig. 13.4 ECG in a patient with acute myocarditis showing ST-segment elevation in the anterior leads and negative T waves in leads V4-6

Myocardial Diseases

Acute myocarditis, which is generally viral in nature, causes electrocardiographic changes that are often hard to distinguish from those associated with acute coronary syndromes. The difficulty is accentuated by the fact that both disorders are associated with chest pain, elevated levels of myocardial-damage markers, and in some cases echocardiographic evidence of segmental wall motion abnormalities. The ECG changes are usually segmental and include upwardly convex ST-segment elevation followed by T-wave inversion (Fig. 13.4).

Electrocardiographic changes indicative of obstructive hypertrophic cardiomyopathy should be analyzed with care because this primary cardiomyopathy is associated with a high risk of sudden death. It should be suspected when the ECG (often being performed for screening purposes alone) reveals left ventricular hypertrophy and T-wave inversion in the anterolateral leads (Fig. 13.5).

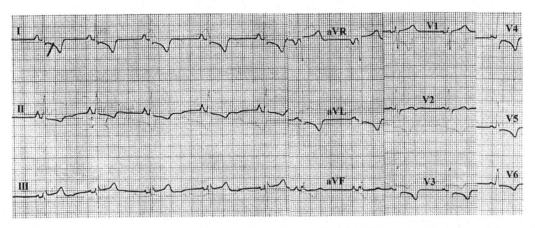

Fig. 13.5 ECG in a patient with obstructive hypertrophic cardiomyopathy. The QRS voltage is increased, and T-wave inversion and ST-segment depression are seen in the anterolateral regions

The Electrocardiogram in Disorders of the Pulmonary Circulation

14

Acute Cor Pulmonale—Pulmonary Embolism

The electrocardiogram (ECG) is a specific but relatively insensitive tool for diagnosing acute cor pulmonale, which is almost always caused by pulmonary embolism. Acute overload of the right ventricle is manifested by a typical triad of ECG features referred to as the $S_1Q_3T_3$ complex or McGinn and White triad. It includes the presence of S waves in lead I and Q waves with T-wave inversion in lead III (Fig. 14.1). Acute cor pulmonale can also be associated with right axis deviation, transient right bundle-branch block (RBBB), and T-wave inversion in the right precordial leads (Fig. 14.2). It has been suggested that inverted T waves in lead V2 or V3 are a common ECG sign of massive pulmonary embolism. In another study on pulmonary embolism, the pseudoinfarction pattern (QR in V1) and T-wave inversion in lead V2 were strongly correlated with the presence of right ventricular dysfunction and independent predictors of an unfavorable clinical outcome.

This ECG picture is generally transient: when the acute phase of the disease has passed, the tracing generally becomes completely normal. The McGinn and White triad is observed only in around 25% of all patients. In the vast majority of cases in which pulmonary embolism is clinically suspected, ECG changes are minimal and may be completely absent.

Large-scale studies have shown that even in the presence of massive pulmonary embolism, the McGinn-White triad, RBBB, right axis deviation and tall, pointed P waves in lead III are found only in about one fourth of all patients. Nonspecific findings that need to be interpreted in light of the clinical findings include sinus tachycardia secondary to hypoxemia and transient, isolated RBBB caused by right ventricular overload. Only 5–10% of patients with pulmonary embolism present right axis deviation, and left axis deviation is actually just as common.

M. Romanò, *Text Atlas of Practical Electrocardiography*,
DOI 10.1007/978-88-470-5741-8_14, © Springer-Verlag Italia 2015

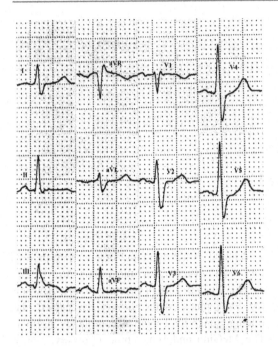

Fig. 14.1 Massive pulmonary embolism: The ECG shows the classic $S_1Q_3T_3$ pattern (McGinn-White triad) and incomplete RBBB

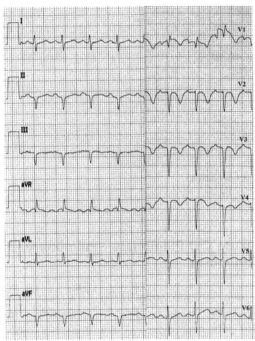

Fig. 14.2 Pulmonary embolism: The most obvious ECG features are the signs of acute right ventricular overload: qR complexes in lead V1 and QS complexes with negative T waves in leads V2 and V3. Exclusion of myocardial ischemia is of fundamental importance in this case

Chronic Cor Pulmonale

Chronic cor pulmonale is characterized by a combination of hypertrophy and dilatation of the right ventricle secondary to pulmonary hypertension (excluding secondary forms caused by congenital heart disease or left-sided heart disease). In these cases, too, the diagnostic sensitivity of the ECG findings is low: it shows signs of enlargement of the right atria and ventricle (Fig. 14.3). The abnormalities are more evident when pressure in the pulmonary vasculature is markedly increased (Fig. 14.4).

Fig. 14.3 Chronic cor pulmonale caused by chronic obstructive pulmonary disease (COPD). The main ECG features include high-voltage P waves in the inferior limb leads (sign of right atrial enlargement), a vertical electrical axis, qR complexes in lead V1 with ST-segment abnormalities suggestive of right ventricular overload

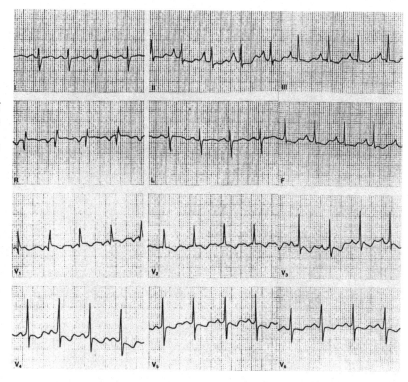

Fig. 14.4 Primary pulmonary hypertension with severe right atrial and ventricular overload in a young women. The ECG shows signs of right atrial and ventricular enlargement, the latter manifested by qR complexes in V1-V3 and ST-segment depression. The electrical axis is also deviated to the right

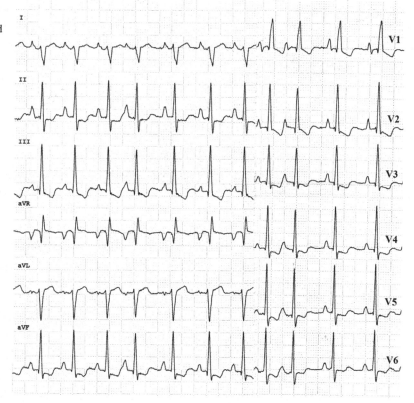

Electrocardiographic Changes Caused by Drugs and Electrolyte Abnormalities

15

Drug-Induced Changes

A number of cardioactive drugs can cause changes in the electrocardiogram (ECG), the antiarrhythmic agents in particular. The most important effects produced by these drugs are bradyarrhythmias, which have been discussed in detail in Chap. 5. In this chapter, we will examine some of the specific effects of individual drugs, with special emphasis on their proarrhythmic effects.

Figure 15.1 illustrates what is referred to as the digitalis effect. It is characterized by typical bowl-shaped depression of the ST segment, sometimes with shortening of the QT interval. These changes reflect the effect of digitalis (even at therapeutic blood levels) on the transmembrane action potential. Another commonly used drug, amiodarone, affects phase 3 of the cardiac action potential, thereby prolonging the QT interval. This is especially common during long-term treatment. The QT interval is sometimes markedly prolonged (Fig. 15.2), and this increases the risk of severe arrhythmias like torsades de pointes (Fig. 15.3). QT-interval prolongation is the most classic proarrhythmic effect of the antiarrhythmic drugs (see also Chap. 6). Iatrogenic arrhythmias related to a prolonged QT interval are also caused by sotalol, a beta-blocker whose effects on phase 3 of the action potential are just as powerful as those of amiodarone (Fig. 15.4). Finally, the Class IC antiarrhythmics, flecainide and propafenone, can produce significant ECG changes. Figure 6.31 shows an ECG recorded during flecainide therapy, which documents the presence of atrial flutter with 1:1 atrioventricular conduction and aberrant QRS morphology. As for propafenone, it causes changes that resemble those of the Brugada syndrome (see Chap. 9): RBBB and ST-segment elevation in leads V1 and V2 (Fig. 15.5). (In this patient, the presence of the genetic syndrome had been excluded.)

Table 9.1 lists the cardioactive drugs that can induce prolongation of the QT interval, sometimes with life-threatening effects. These drugs should always be considered when faced with unexplained prolongation of the QT interval.

M. Romanò, *Text Atlas of Practical Electrocardiography*,
DOI 10.1007/978-88-470-5741-8_15, © Springer-Verlag Italia 2015

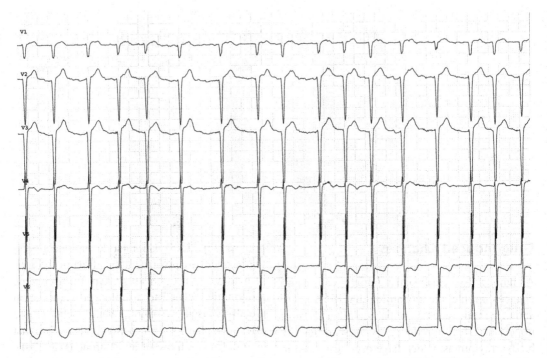

Fig. 15.1 The ST segment displays bowl-shaped depression (especially evident in lead V6), which is typical of the digitalis effect. Atrial fibrillation is also present

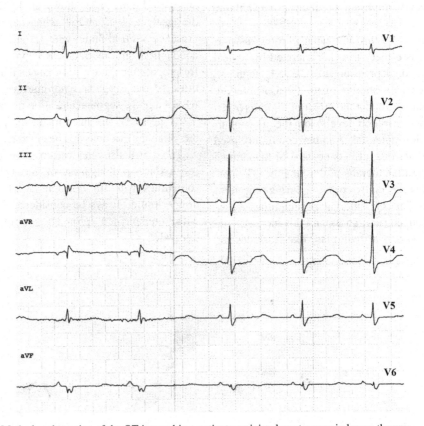

Fig. 15.2 Marked prolongation of the QT interval in a patient receiving long-term amiodarone therapy

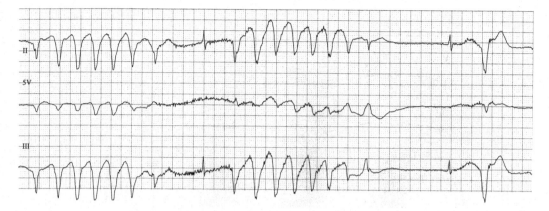

Fig. 15.3 Cardiac monitor strip showing recurrent torsade de pointes ventricular tachycardia in a patient with marked prolongation of the QT interval secondary to chronic use of amiodarone

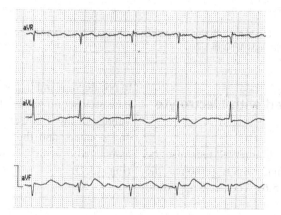

Fig. 15.4 Atrial flutter with variable atrioventricular conduction associated with sotalol-induced lengthening of the QT interval

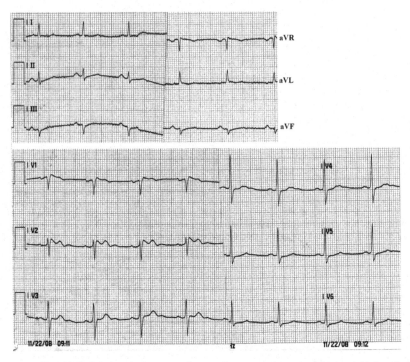

Fig. 15.5 Brugada-like ECG changes during propafenone therapy characterized by a right bundle-branch block (RBBB) and ST elevation in leads V1 and V2

Changes Associated with Electrolyte Abnormalities

Lengthening of the QT interval can also be causes by hypokalemia, which prolongs the action potential (Fig. 15.6). The same applies to hypocalcemia and hypomagnesemia. In contrast, increased serum levels of potassium increase the voltage of the T waves, which thus become tall and pointed, and these changes are frequently associated with conduction disturbances (Fig. 15.7).

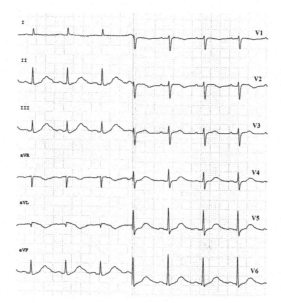

Fig. 15.6 Hypokalemia-induced lengthening of the QT interval

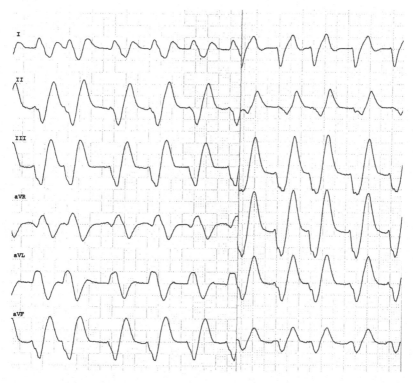

Fig. 15.7 Patient with hyperkalemia (9 mEq/L). The ECG shows tall, pointed T waves in the precordial leads and an associated left bundle-branch block

Brief Bibliography

Antzelevitch C, Brugada P, Borggrefe M et al (2005) Brugada Syndrome: report of the second consensus conference: endorsed by the Heart Rhythm Society and the European Heart Rhythm Association. Circulation 111(5):659–670

Arruda MS, McClelland JH, Wang X et al (1998) Development and validation of an ECG algorithm for identifying accessory pathway ablation site in Wolff-Parkinson-White syndrome. J Cardiovasc Electrophysiol 9(1):2–12

Barrabés JA, Figueras J, Mource C et al (2003) Prognostic value of lead aVR in patients with a first non-ST-segment elevation acute myocardial infarction. Circulation 108(7):814–819

Bayés De Luna A, Wagner G, Birnbaum Y et al (2006) A new terminology for left ventricular walls and location of myocardial infarcts that present Q wave based on the standard of cardiac magnetic resonance imaging: a statement for healthcare professionals from a committee appointed by the International Society for Holter and Noninvasive Electrocardiography. Circulation 114(16):1755–1760

Brugada P, Brugada J, Mont L et al (1991) A new approach to the differential diagnosis of a regular tachycardia with a wide QRS complex. Circulation 83(5):1649–1659

Cerqueira MD, Weissman NJ, Dilsizian V et al (2002) Standardized myocardial segmentation and nomenclature for tomographic imaging of the heart: a statement for healthcare professionals from the Cardiac Imaging Committee of the Council on Clinical Cardiology of the American Heart Association. Circulation 105(4): 539–542

Coumel P, Attuel P, Leclercq JF (1979) Permanent form of junctional reciprocating tachycardia: mechanism, clinical and therapeutic implications. In: Narula OS (ed) Cardiac arrhythmias: electrophysiology, diagnosis and management. Williams and Wilkins, Baltimore

Furman S, Hayes D, Holmes D (1986) A practice of cardiac pacing. Futura Publ. Co., Mt. Kisco, New York

Goldberger E (1942) A simple, indifferent electrocardiographic electrode of zero potential and a technique of obtaining augmented, unipolar, extremity leads. Am Heart J 23:483

Green JS (2005) ECG signs of ischemia & infarction: a story of ST-T and Q-Waves. Power Point presentation. http://jsgreen.tamu.edu

Josephson ME, Wellens HJ (1997) Electrophysiologic evaluation of supraventricular tachycardia. Cardiol Clin 15(4):567–586

Katritsis DG, Camm AJ (2006) Classification and differential diagnosis of atrioventricular nodal reentrant tachycardia. Europace 8(1):29–36

Kenigsberg DN, Khanal S, Kowalski M, Krishnan SC (2007) Prolongation of the QTc interval is seen uniformly during early transmural ischemia. J Am Coll Cardiol 49(12):1299–1305

Kindwall KE, Brown J, Josephson ME (1988) Electrocardiographic criteria for ventricular tachycardia in wide complex left bundle branch block morphology tachycardias. Am J Cardiol 61(15):1279–1283

Medeiros-Domingo A, Iturralde-Torres P, Ackerman MJ (2007) Clinical and genetic characteristics of long QT syndrome. Rev Esp Cardiol 60(7):739–752

Okin PM, Roman MJ, Devereux RB, Kligfield P (1995) Electrocardiographic identification of increased left ventricular mass by simple voltage-duration products. J Am Coll Cardiol 25(2):417–423

Pfister RC, Hutter AM Jr, Newhouse JH (1983) Contrast-medium-induced electrocardiographic abnormalities: comparison of bolus and infusion of methylglucamine iodamide and methylglucamine/sodium diatrizoate. AJR Am J Roentgenol 140(1):149–153

Riva SI, Della Bella P, Fassini G et al (1996) Value of analysis of ST segment changes during tachycardia in determining type of narrow QRS complex tachycardia. J Am Coll Cardiol 27(6):1480–1485

Roden DM (2008) Clinical practice. Long-QT syndrome. N Engl J Med 358(2):169–176

Saoudi N, Cosìo F, Waldo A et al (2001) A classification of atrial flutter and regular atrial tachycardia according to electrophysiological mechanisms and anatomical bases; a Statement from a Joint Expert Group from The Working Group of Arrhythmias of the European Society of Cardiology and the North American Society of Pacing and Electrophysiology. Eur Heart J 22(14): 1162–1182

Schimpf R, Wolpert C, Gaita F et al (2005) Short QT syndrome. Cardiovasc Res 67(3):357–366

M. Romanò, *Text Atlas of Practical Electrocardiography*,
DOI 10.1007/978-88-470-5741-8, © Springer-Verlag Italia 2015

Sgarbossa EB, Pinski SL, Barbagelata A et al (1996) Electrocardiographic diagnosis of evolving acute myocardial infarction in the presence of left bundle-branch block. GUSTO-1 (Global Utilization of Streptokinase and Tissue Plasminogen Activator for Occluded Coronary Arteries) Investigators. N Engl J Med 334(8): 481–487

Slavich G (1997) Elettrocardiografia clinica. Collana: Anestesia e Medicina Critica. Capitolo 2, 316 pagg., Springer-Verlag Italia, Milano

Sodi Pallares D, Medrano G, Bisteni A, Ponce de Leon J (1987) Elettrocardiografia deduttiva e poliparametrica. Il Pensiero Scientifico Editore, Torino

Vereckei A, Duray G, Szénàsi G et al (2007) Application of a new algorithm in the differential diagnosis of wide QRS complex tachycardia. Eur Heart J 28(5): 589–600

Wilson FN et al (1933) The distribution of the action current produced by heart muscle and other excitable tissues immersed in extensive conducting media. J Gen Physiol 16:423

Zimetbaum PJ, Josephson ME (2003) Use of the electrocardiogram in acute myocardial infarction. N Engl J Med 348(10):933–940